To Sandy,

A woman is her head on straight & we're workin

IS YOUR HEAD ON STRAIGHT?

to keep it there.

A New Approach for Healing Head Trauma

Dr. Patrick Gallagher

Is Your Head on Straight? A New Approach for Healing Head Trauma
©2017 by Dr. Patrick Gallagher
chiropracticfirstnc.com

ISBN: 978-0-9989353-0-0
Library of Congress Control Number: 2017910730

The publisher has strived to be as accurate and complete as possible in the creation of this book.

Warning and Disclaimer

The information in this book is published in good faith and for general information purposes only. The author and publisher do not make any warranties about the information contained in this book. The information is designed to provide helpful information on the subjects discussed.

This book is not meant to be used, nor should it be used, to diagnose or treat any medical condition. The diagnosis or treatment of any medical problem should be handled by the reader's personal physician. Any action taken by the reader regarding the information contained in this book is strictly at the reader's own risk. Neither the author nor the publisher will be liable for any damages or losses sustained by the reader in connection with the use of the information contained in this book.

While all attempts have been made to verify information provided for this publication, the publisher assumes no responsibility for errors, omissions, or contrary interpretation of the subject matter herein. Any perceived slights of specific persons, peoples, or organizations are unintended.

Printed in USA by Dr. Patrick Gallagher

Dedication

I would like to dedicate this book to one individual and two groups of people. First off, to Dr. Roy W. Sweat: if it were not for him, this book would not have come to pass. It took his lifetime dedication to studying the upper cervical area to unlock the secret that enables some six hundred doctors to now perform miracles in the lives of the truly hurting.

Next I would like to dedicate this book to my patients, who trusted me as their doctor and without whom I never would have had anything to write about. It was the stories of how they now enjoy life—with their heads back on straight—that inspired me to put pen to paper.

Lastly, I also would like to dedicate my first book to all those who read it and take action—for those who find hope in these pages that their lives of misery or dependence on pain pills for normalcy may have a happy ending after all. This book is dedicated to the hope that they, too, can have their heads put back on straight and live out a blessed life.

To find a board certified atlas orthogonalist near you, visit **http://globalao.com**.

For Eastern North Carolina, visit Dr. Gallagher's website, **http://chiropracticfirstnc.com**.

Contents

Foreword

By Dr. Roy W. Sweat

Dr. Gallagher is a peculiar Board Certified Atlas Orthogonal (BCAO) chiropractor because he treats some of the most unusual cases. I have even shared some unique cases from his clinics in my seminars. One such case involved a patient who had his skull crushed in. As a result, the alignment of his head was way off-center (13 mm), yet Dr. Gallagher, applying what I taught him, re-centered his head to within 1 mm! Dr. Gallagher seems to have an uncanny knack for attracting truly challenging cases. He presents a number of those in this book, *Is Your Head on Straight?* It takes a gift to treat those who are truly traumatized, to look past their pain and symptoms and see what is really going on.

I am so glad that a BCAO doctor has found the time to present our unique discipline of care in a reader-friendly work. I often stress at Advance AO seminars that doctors need to reach out to other health care providers to strive to educate them about our line of work. Now, Dr. Gallagher has written a book that explains in detail what we do, how we do it, and why we do it—providing a dozen or so case studies as examples of some of the results he has seen in his clinics.

Apart from other health care providers, his writing is also geared toward the lay reader, the patient or family member of a patient who has tried the medical route for relief and is still dealing with discomfort. Evident in his subtitle, "A New Approach to Healing from Traumas to the Head," this is a book that aims to be a beacon of hope to those who suffer. Although I invented the

Atlas Orthogonal Percussion Instrument that Dr. Gallagher references almost fifty years ago, if readers have never heard about it, then it's new to them. Dr. Gallagher does a good job showing readers just how far-reaching the results of the atlas orthogonal (AO) technique can be and how many people it could help. Hopefully his writing will show readers how important it is to have your atlas checked to make sure your head is on straight.

To the reader who is pondering this book, you are holding in your hands a well-written testament to how one person's life went through so much trauma, yet came out upright at the end. The unique approach to giving relief at the base of the skull is something I helped developed a half century ago. Now, at ninety years old, it puts a huge smile on my face knowing that this information will get into the hands of many people that could benefit from that knowledge.

I know the difficulty of trying to get the atlas orthogonal technique utilized in a clinical setting. I am more worried by the doctors who don't call me than those who do. We hear from Dr. Gallagher about every month and a half with a unique case, seeking advice about how to better treat his patients.

A final note: Although I think Dr. Gallagher is crazy for running all those marathons, we're proud of him for the work he is doing on some truly difficult cases and the results he is getting.

Acknowledgments

First off, thanks be to God, who through His divine wisdom brought good out of the mistakes of my life. Thanks to the Sweats, Dr. Roy, Dr. Matthew, and Tecla, who have been an extended family for me and were essential to providing some of the materials for this book.

Thanks to Margaret Baddour ("Teach"), who taught me to show but not tell and to believe I could put this book together. Equally, Susan Bowmer, who worked many late nights with me "working the words." Thanks to the Goldsboro Writers Group who corporately kept me grounded to make this writing for the lay person. Thanks to Diana M. Needham, who knows just how to orchestrate all the activities required to publish a book. Thanks to my family for helping me through a difficult part of my life. To my dad who advised me to seek out chiropractic care thirty seven years ago and also for his help in editing my book. To my mom, who was always there to help me find a better way to say what was bottled up inside. To Drs. Bill Macchi and Florence Licata, thanks for sharing your knowledge and insight. Thanks to my wife, Blondine for her love through it all. And to all the others who helped me shape up this ten-year idea for sharing something that many know nothing about.

Introduction

Is Your Head on Straight?

I remember riding my friend's yellow Suzuki 80 motorcycle up the hill to check out who was approaching our party. Being the host of this keg party in the field, I felt it was my duty to check on all newcomers, especially female ones. Discovering it was just my sister Elaine and her friend Cheryl, I turned around and headed back to the party. The next thing I recall I am seated upstairs in the back porch of our home, facing those very fields and my mother is feeding me through a straw, just as she had when I was one year old.

It's May of 1980 and I am seventeen years old. My mom is feeding me because my jaws are wired shut. Not only does my mouth not work, my brain is not firing too well ether. I feel as if I had been dragged 100 yards through a cornfield by a spooked stallion. How did I get here?

Indeed, my head was not on straight, which was just one of the severe injuries from that motorcycle accident. My life changed forever in a split second, and I began a difficult journey back to health. Many on this same journey hit lots of dead ends that could possibly be avoided. One thing I know for sure: If pharmaceutical companies are your guides to a path of recovery, you may not be a happy camper at the end of the trail.

Having the experience of being a patient who was traumatized both physically and emotionally from a motorcycle accident while witnessing the impacts not only to me but also to my family, I've learned firsthand what works and what doesn't.

This book is written not only from the real-world experience of the injured patient but also from the perspective of a specialized doctor who focuses on correcting the area where the skull meets the neck. Profound, miraculous results have been created with patients whose cases were written off by other medical providers.

As a highly trained atlas orthogonalist chiropractor, I address a unique insult (i.e., an injury or interference to the normal function of the body) to the nervous system that is brought on when your head is off-center. When that insult is removed, it is amazing to see how miraculously the body can and does heal. I am grateful to call the inventor of this special technique, Dr. Roy W. Sweat, a great friend.

In these pages, you will learn about this special technique that only six hundred of the approximately sixty thousand chiropractors worldwide are certified to apply. Being one of those six hundred is why I am passionate about writing this book and the results we see in our clinic. Although not practiced by many, the technique, called atlas orthogonal (AO), is respected by other chiropractors. Within these pages, I share the testimony, among others, of the wife of a chiropractor that does not practice AO but she travels almost two hours one way to come to my clinic to receive this life-changing care. I have been applying this procedure for the past seventeen years on a wide variety of patients with symptoms ranging from nauseating migraines to those with vertigo so severe that their world is spinning out of control before their very eyes. Many have even encouraged me to write this very book, to share how this special procedure helped them to regain normal function. They are thrilled to share how that light tap, just behind their ear, rocked their world for the better as their health returned naturally.

The truth is we don't know what we don't know. Within these pages you'll encounter the concept of "innate intelligence," the body's instinctual attempt to adapt for a better life. The doctor within needs to be heard and worked with—not against! We are naturally designed by our Creator to be self-healing beings. We don't always need parts removed or chemicals added to be well and healthy. Dorland's Medical Dictionary, a widely respected source in the medical profession, defines *health* as "a condition of optimum physical, social, mental and spiritual wellbeing— not merely the absence of disease or infirmities."[1] In line with that I will show that a person's health can and should be a natural process of functioning the way we were created to.

If you or someone you care about is suffering from symptoms tied to the head not being properly aligned, this book is for you. Did you know that aside from the dozen cranial nerves, which exit through different openings in your skull, essentially all other nerve function goes out the *foramen magnum*? That's Latin for the *large opening* located at the base of your skull. Yet right under that opening is a most extraordinary bone of the spine called the atlas. It does so much, yet it is the smallest bone in your spine. Not only is it the lightest bone in the spine, it is the most mobile one, and when it is not where it belongs your nervous system can be greatly challenged. Beyond vertigo and migraine headaches the symptoms can be quite varied; yet one overriding complaint is a pain or discomfort where the skull meets the neck.

If you long for a way to have things restored to normal in your life or that of a loved one where there is a history of a trauma, then the answer may well lie within this book.

---

[1] *Dorland's Illustrated Medical Dictionary*, 32nd ed. (Philadelphia, PA: Elsevier, 2012).

A Special Bonus Gift from Dr. Gallagher

Now that you've secured your copy of *Is Your Head on Straight?* you are on your way to learning about a very important yet often overlooked disturbance to your nervous system. Not only will you encounter numerous cases of patients who suffered from neurological insult but you will also discover their miraculous stories of regaining a balanced life.

There are so many drugs to mask the pain of migraines, vertigo, and other ailments, but if the atlas is out of proper alignment, medicine cannot correct the problem. When you finish this book, not only will you know what symptoms are common indicators of this type of injury but you'll also know how to seek the care to correct the problem.

To thank you for your purchase, I have created a special feature with ten tips for a healthier spine. Please visit the following URL and tell us where to send this bonus gift:

http://isyourheadonstraightbook.com/bonus

I am in your corner. Let me know if I can help further.

Here's to getting your or your loved one's head back on straight!

Sincerely yours in the world's greatest health profession,

Patrick Gallagher, DC, BC, AO

Patrick Gallagher, DC, BCAO
http://chiropracticfirstnc.com

PART I

From Patient to Doctor

Chapter One

How I Spent My Summer Vacation in 1980

It is summer 1980. School is out! Hallelujah! I made it through my junior year of high school and am now officially a senior! The sun is shining. The landscape has just turned green in the Mid-Hudson Valley in Poughkeepsie, New York. The beer is cold. There's nothing to do but enjoy the day. My buddies and I are ready to *PARTY!* The first kegger of the season has officially begun.

Okay, so at seventeen we are a bit too young to be legally throwing a kegger. However, my friend Dave, an older man of eighteen, was able to pick up a keg and bring it to the party.

The party site, a former cornfield long overgrown, is about 150 yards from end to end with a small valley in the middle. It is located 200 yards behind my family's house. No one is close enough to complain about a bunch of high school kids celebrating the end of the school year and the beginning of summer.

Some of my friends have their lives mapped out. They plan to graduate from high school at eighteen, go to college, graduate from college at twenty-two, immediately launch their careers, marry at twenty-four, have their first child by twenty-eight, and retire by fifty. Well, good luck with all that. I have no ambitions or plans, just my buddies Jeff and Dave, fishing and camping in the Catskills. I have no game plan beyond my day-to-day existence. I am just going through the motions as a teenager.

I remember about eight of us guys and a couple of girls, including my younger sister Karen, were already celebrating when I saw two more girls coming down from the far corner of the field to join us. An oval trail borders the field, so you can walk or ride to any part of it.

As a red-blooded American teenaged boy, it is my prerogative—no, my obligation, my responsibility—to check out any and all incoming females. One of my friends has a yellow Suzuki 80 motorcycle and I hop onto it to see who's coming to join our party.

I don't bother putting on a helmet (although Dave still claims they were all yelling at me to do so). Why should I? I'm just riding across the field. Who needs a helmet to go that far? About three-quarters of the way across the field I see that it's only my older sister Elaine and her friend Cheryl, so I turn around and head back to the party. Turning around and heading back down the hill—that's all I remember.

Maybe I hit a woodchuck hole or simply lost control and jackknifed, but suddenly I was airborne!

The bike and I land about fifteen feet apart. My body hits like a burlap sack full of sand and folds to the left. The left side of my skull strikes the ground first, as evidenced by the fractured left jaw, the force of the impact compounded by the weight of the rest of my body. This forms a whipping motion to the left so forceful that I fracture some ribs on my left and misalign my spine from left to right. The impact is so dynamic that my Jell-O-like brain is rattled unconscious. Here is where physics comes into play: F = M x A (*force* equals *mass* times *acceleration*). The mass of my body traveling through space came to an abrupt stop in milliseconds, and the force of the impact challenged the integrity of my body like never before in my life.

This causes a definite change in the partying atmosphere. The keg is abandoned as everyone runs to the crash scene.

Elaine and Cheryl reach me first. There must have already been blood trickling from my mouth due to the impact of my lips on my braces. Cheryl takes it upon herself to try to bring me around by picking me up by the collar and slapping my face. Not a good thing to do under the circumstances, but we are kids and this is common practice on television. Of course, the people on television are actors and stuntmen, not accident victims gushing real blood and suffering life-threatening injuries. Dave rushes to me and sees my eyelids fluttering and eyeballs rolling to the back of my head. Karen runs home to call 911 and the call is dispatched to the Rochdale fire department. An ambulance is dispatched while the fire department directs them with the best route to get to me.

The fire department knows the area pretty well and quickly decides the best route is to come in from the back of the field, about 150 yards from the crash site. A creek and tree line separate us from them, yet their four-wheeled rescue vehicle crosses the creek and chainsaws drop trees, allowing the ambulance to come through to me.

It takes about twenty or thirty minutes for them to reach us. It feels like a lifetime for my friends and family. I am still blissfully unconscious.

Dave remembers: Patrick was riding back to us when he hit a chuck hole; the field was full of them, and crashed. At first, I thought he was monkeying with us. We were terrified! No one knew what to do! People were screaming and Patrick's little sister Karen ran home to get help.

Dad remembers: Patrick was first picked up by the fire-and-rescue vehicle, which then transferred him to the ambulance. I received a phone call saying Patrick had been in a motorcycle accident and was being taken to St. Francis Hospital in downtown Poughkeepsie, New York. Racing to the accident site, I saw an ambulance with its lights flashing and sirens screaming heading from our home and followed it. Fortunately, I guessed correctly. Yes, it was my son unconscious in the back of the ambulance.

The hospital was run by very nice nuns who said the first good sign was that Patrick responded to having a needle stuck into his foot.

Everybody was frantic. Of the five children in our family, if anything could happen to any one of them, it would happen to Patrick. Patrick was born with a collapsed lung. The doctors would not even tell Mary whether she had a boy or a girl until they were sure he would live. Patrick was baptized immediately in case he died, as was the standard for the Catholic hospital. "He's gonna' be a fighter," one of the nuns said.

Patrick pulled through but had plenty of other near misses. As a two-year-old toddling across the living room, he fell and hit his face on the coffee table. We cleaned up the blood and put cold cloths on his face. Later that night, I went to check on him and found his sheets covered in blood. It turns out he had not only hurt his face but had also bitten through his tongue. He had been drinking his own blood up to that point and now it was trickling out onto his sheets. We rushed him to the emergency room where they could not numb his tongue as they were stitching it up, and his screams could be heard throughout the hospital.

While in the hospital after the motorcycle accident, it was touch-and-go for eleven very long days, for Patrick was in a coma. The prognosis was not good. There was not much hope that Patrick would survive; if he did, there was a very real possibility of his remaining in a vegetative state for the rest of his life. The neurosurgeon was only concerned with the injury to Patrick's head. He told us Patrick would never remember the accident and he does not.

They had to re-break his jaw as it had started healing while he was in the coma, yet it had to be realigned. For some reason, they opted not to operate on his jaw while he was still in a coma. When Patrick finally woke up, he had to re-learn how to speak and talk with a broken jaw.

Mom remembers: I had been out with a friend and got the news when I returned home. One of my daughters told me what happened and that he had been taken to St. Francis Hospital. I immediately drove there and found Patrick unconscious and bandaged. After being there awhile with the rest of the family, I began to cry and a nun came up to comfort me and said, "I'm glad to see you cry. It's good for you."

TAKE AWAY: NO MATTER WHAT YOU'RE DRIVING, DON'T DRINK AND DRIVE.

Chapter Two

Coming Back Around

I spend the next eleven days in a coma and nearly an entire month in St. Francis Hospital.

With so many critical injuries, the doctors have a tough time deciding where to start. The jaw and spine are obvious, but they can't account for what appears to be internal bleeding. Through their testing they can see that I have a pool of blood in my abdomen, yet they don't know how it got there. They poke holes in my abdomen to try to find the source then realize the "full bird cage" of silver braces on my teeth has done such a job on my lips that I have been swallowing my own blood, like I did at the age of two.

Once I regain consciousness, they put me back under to re-break the left side of my jaw. They use my braces to wire my mouth shut. For the next two months, everything I eat comes through a straw. Later I graduate to food, which Mom remembers processing through a blender and feeding me. Mom also helped me recall words and encouraged me to be ready to continue my schooling. She now feels this experience of healing brought us closer.

As for my mental capacity, that was definitely a process in the making. I had to re-learn a lot of basic things, like speech and reasoning, in addition to my motor skills being challenged. I would ask the hospital staff, "Waz y'all gonna do to me?" with a deep Southern accent rarely heard in Poughkeepsie, New York. I was raised in Huntsville, Alabama, from age one to eleven. As my brain began to heal, it drew upon that portion of my early memory for the speech process.

I am unsure if it was a side effect of the medicine or a reaction to the traumatic brain injury (TBI), but I began having suicidal tendencies. Once, while deep-sea fishing off the New Jersey coast, I told my father to "hold onto me—I may jump overboard." Another time, I told him I had the urge to step into oncoming traffic. I can only conjecture, but I sense that after so close a brush with death, the possibility of being there stirred something within. This went on for about half a year after the accident.

My recovery was filled with pain; the route to recovery prescribed to me was to take muscle relaxers and pain pills as I felt was needed, and boy did I need something! I hurt over my whole body. But even at seventeen, I instinctively knew I was not happy with the way we were proceeding in the effort to get my body back to the way it once was. It was this dissatisfaction that pushed me to explore different paths for seeking relief. Eventually, it was the chest pain I had with every deep breath that led me to take my father's advice and seek a chiropractor. My father had been to a chiropractor and was aware of the benefits of that type of therapy.

The first chiropractor I went to was a large but gentle man with a warm smile and a firm handshake by the name of Lester Lutz, Doctor of Chiropractic (DC). Upon taking some X-rays, he informed me that my chest pain was caused by fractured ribs on my left side. The hospital must have taken X-rays of that area, but sometimes it takes days or even weeks for a subtle fracture to show up on such scans. The fracture sites are often only found after new bone starts forming. Dr. Lutz began making corrections to realign my body. Under his care, my body began to function better, with much less stress on my skeletal structure.

Through this ordeal, I am introduced to chiropractic care and am impressed by the whole science and logic of it. I learned that our bodies are built with a definite design and pattern and deviations from that pattern are not good, period. With the force of that motorcycle accident acting upon my seventeen-year-old frame, I was definitely in need of massive realigning.

Dr. Lutz was a very caring and passionate man who inspired me with his chiropractic success stories, especially that of my own. He took a liking to me from the beginning. He understood what I had been through in the accident and continued to work with my light, 155-pound frame to bring me back into structural alignment. I found that a lot of my full-body pains were lessened with just a few corrective adjustments.

It was just before Christmas in my senior year of high school when I knew, without a doubt, that with God's help I was going to become a chiropractor. Immediately after high school I enrolled in Duchess Community College, in Poughkeepsie. Two years later, I enrolled in Life Chiropractic College, now named Life University, located in Marietta, Georgia.

TAKE AWAY: DON'T SETTLE FOR LESS. IF YOUR BODY IS COMPLAINING, STRIVE TO FIND OUT WHAT THE PROBLEM IS.

Chapter Three

Got My Soul on Straight

I was a cradle Catholic. My aunt was a nun and the principal of a very prominent Catholic school in New Jersey. Going to church as a family was something we just did, no question about it. Growing up, I was active in the church because I liked being involved. I was even an altar boy. I liked the special attire, ringing the bell and the attention and respect the position afforded. I took my religious beliefs at face value. I never questioned any of it. It was just the way it was. Sunday was church day just as it was also the day for football games in the fall. As a child and young adult, I saw nothing more to religion than that it was what was done.

I had moved away from home for the first time in my life, and now here I was, at the age of twenty, off at college. It was October 5, 1983, my second day on campus at Life Chiropractic College in Marietta, Georgia. I stop by the Morale House, where all the student activities happen. That night, they were hosting an information session for all the different clubs and activities on campus. There must have been a dozen or more clubs represented.

Life College is noted for training students in the many different chiropractic techniques for adjusting the spine, and members from each discipline were represented. There were also some sororities and fraternities at the information session. What catches my eye is a drop-dead-gorgeous brunette sitting at a table representing the Christian Fellowship Club (CFC).

I quickly make my way over to her table. I start a conversation with her just to make small talk, yet I can see in her eyes and hear in her voice that this woman knows something that I don't.

I begin with a disconnect: Why is there a group that meets Thursday nights to discuss what you always discuss on Sundays? I tell her I have always gone to church; it's just what we did as a family. I share with her my accolades as a child: communion, confession, confirmation, and, of course, I stick in my altar boy stint too. After a lively conversation that lasted probably ten to fifteen minutes in which I tried to defend my stance that following tradition was a way to get into heaven, what stood out to me was her statement: "You can have a personal relationship with Jesus." That was something new to me. Although I was sure that phrase lay in the doctrine of Catholicism, in my advanced life of twenty years, I didn't recall hearing that or noting any importance placed upon that concept. The concept of having a personal relationship with this historic Jesus, who I had known of my entire life, stuck with me like an unearthed treasure chest, a huge "Ah-ha!" was about to unfold upon me and rock my world like never before.

Mary, the brunette, gives me a tract called the Road Map to Heaven. Her husband is also a student, with less than a year to go, who will later become my treating student clinician. He was the current president of the CFC, so it made perfect sense that his wife would help recruit new members. God used her to catch my eye and led me to see things that I didn't even know I was seeking. Little did I know then that I would become president of that very club in my last year and a half at Life.

During my conversation with Mary, we disagreed on some points. I thought I knew God, but after talking with her the certainty of my attitude toward that knowledge was shaken. That night, I stood in front of my bathroom mirror praying: "God, I think I know You, but if I don't, I want to know You." God saw the sincerity of my heart. Here I was, a very young man, out on his

ROAD MAP TO HEAVEN

1) WHO HAS SINNED?

"For all have sinned and come short of the glory of God."   Romans 3:23

2) WHAT IS THE PENALTY FOR SIN?

"The wages of sin is death; but the free gift of God is eternal life through Jesus Christ our Lord." Romans 6:23

3) HOW MAY I BE SAVED?

"For whosoever shall call upon the name of the Lord shall be saved."   Romans 10:13

4) WHAT HAPPENS WHEN I ASK CHRIST TO SAVE ME?

"Behold, I stand at the door and knock; if any man hear my voice and open the door, I will come in and fellowship with him and he with me."   Revelation 3:20

5) HOW DO I ASK CHRIST TO SAVE ME?

Dear Lord Jesus, I admit that I am a sinner. I believe that you died for me and paid the penalty for my sins. I need your forgiveness and I am willing to turn from my sins. I open the door of my heart and invite you to enter my life as my personal Saviour. I am willing to follow and obey you as the Lord of my life.

You should pray this prayer right now if it expresses the conviction of your heart.

This is the very tract I received October 5, 1983.

own for the first time, open for change. I guess I was "low hanging fruit" needing to be harvested, for I was still wild on the vine.

The previous Saturday night I had been at Baby Does, a hot nightspot north of Atlanta. There I had met and danced the night away with a really nice girl. Upon saying good night, she had given me her number twice, but I didn't write it down, telling her I had a "super memory."

Wrong! I must have tried four or five different numbers before conceding the fact that my memory was not as good as I had led her to believe. In the big scheme of things, I think God intervened, knowing I was due for a much more enduring relationship to begin three nights later at the information session. Had I started a hot new relationship the previous weekend, I don't know how attuned I would have been to my true spiritual need. As in other relationships, my thoughts would have been on the girl and how our relationship was shaping up. Yet, I was spiritually dead, and God, through Mary, was going to breathe life into my spiritually lifeless soul.

With a new hunger for God and His word, I began attending a Pentecostal church. One Sunday the preacher was speaking on the importance and meaning of baptism. I knew I had already been baptized a number of times. Twice as a baby: once at the hospital with the collapsed lung and then again months later at a Catholic Mass, and again as a seventeen-year-old in a coma. Now I knew what it was all about. I would not be the passive recipient of my next baptism, but the seeker compelled to follow God's word and be baptized. I gained a new understanding of the change within and that the outward presentation of a baptism is a presentation of an inward change.

Joyce Faircloth, the leader of CFC, baptized me at my church, Marietta Church of God, on Thursday, April 12, 1984.

I recall one Thursday evening at the CFC earlier that year with clarity. I was still new in the group and reveling at the changes in my life: I had a hunger for the Word of God; I desired to go to church not out of an act of obedience but a desire to know my God all the more. Our group was not too large; we probably averaged five or six students. We met in a classroom module on a hill. Fortunately, it was uphill and upwind from our cadaver lab, with its nauseating formaldehyde odor. Toward the end of the meetings we went over prayer request and needs. In that meeting, Joyce prayed over Tom as he knelt, desiring the gift of "speaking in tongues." As members, we laid hands on him in agreement. I was standing to Tom's left, and for some reason Joyce took her hands off of Tom and placed them on my shoulders. I sank to my knees as she prayed.

I began to feel warmth build up in my chest, and I uttered my first word in an unknown language. I was awash in tears of gratitude for God's hand and favor in visiting me. At first only one or two words came to me, yet that increased until I was having an ongoing dialog with pitch, body language, connotation, tone, and emphasis. I even sang in the spirit with my new gift, speaking in tongues.

As I prayed and spoke in this language, a peace flowed over me. My shoulders dropped and a smile rose on my face. I entered an arena in which I could never speak a word out of place. It was not me choosing the words I spoke; they were only what my newly saved soul, in communion with its Creator, desired. Often I did not receive an interpretation of that blissful dialogue. I simply had the peace of having just communed with the Creator in exactly the way He wanted the talk to go. There were times when, if I listened within, He would give me an interpretation of what had flowed out of me. It was only one word at a time. It was nothing profound or earth rattling, simply His Word or intent brought to light. It was specific to me in where I was or what I was going through. With that Word or enlightenment, the journey in this life became that much more bearable.

Now that I had come to this new understanding, I was rethinking life. Should I step out in this new reality and pursue a calling to serve God? I remember exactly where I was when I got my answer. It wasn't too far from the module where the CFC met. It was behind the student clinic on a narrow stretch of ground bordered by a tree-lined fence, a handy place in which to find some space alone.

I sat down on the grass and felt the warm Georgia sun on my face, and then I got really quiet and prayed: "God, are You calling me to a pastoral position or evangelism? A few close friends at school are suggesting I seem to be very passionate about my faith and might want to consider a track in that direction." One thing I learned early on about praying was that it sure helps to be sincere in your prayer life, for He knows our intentions better than we could ever hope to. Granting the assurance I needed, He spoke to my soul: "I have a plan and purpose for you, and it is in line with becoming a doctor of chiropractic." That was all I needed to hear. With that affirmation, I got up off the grass and pushed through the academic requirements to become a chiropractic doctor.

Fast forward to 2017: Since that life-changing Tuesday night when I met Mary and was awakened to the possibility of having a personal relationship with God, I have had a hunger for God and His Word. I read the Bible almost daily. When traveling on Sundays, I find churches to attend. I take active positions in my home church and have helped lead people to the Lord. I still have and follow the Road Map to Heaven that Mary gave me that crucial night at Life Chiropractic College.

TAKE AWAY: HAVE A PERSONAL RELATIONSHIP WITH JESUS CHRIST. LIFE IS TOUGH ENOUGH BY ITSELF, AND IT IS MEANINGLESS WITHOUT HIM.

Chapter Four

Life Goes On

After that spiritual and eternal life change, little did I know I was in for another life-altering event. There was a buzz on campus about the upper cervical chiropractors who put 90 percent of their focus on adjusting only one bone. This caught my interest. Why just one bone? As God would have it, I met and became a patient of the president of the Life Upper Cervical Club, Frank Falowski. His stories of the work he, as a student clinician, had already seen inspired me twofold, both as a patient and as a student. As I shared the stories of my motorcycle wreck with the soon-to-be-graduate Dr. Falowski, he gave me hope that I would be a good candidate for this care. If that type of care could improve my life, all the more reason to get a jump on learning this way of helping my future patients.

It did not take much convincing on my part, since I had already chosen to become a chiropractor and had received enough care to commit my life to practicing chiropractic. It was agreed that Frank would take me under his care. He was the first chiropractor to introduce me to the reality of having your head put back on straight via adjusting the atlas. The very next day I became his student patient. X-rays confirmed what he had said, that one bone was, sure enough, pushed up to the right side of my skull and twisted backward.

With that atlas deviation, my right leg was compensating by pulling up a half inch; this was my body's attempt to deal with the misalignment. This was measured as I was lying on my back.

When I sat up, Frank felt the top of my neck just underneath my skull, and he found four different tender spots, two per side. He then had me lay on my left side with my head on a B.J. side posture toggle table, which is a chiropractic table with a special headpiece where the head lies. When pressure is applied to it, the headpiece drops down about a quarter of an inch, allowing the doctor's hands to be off the spine.

He rolled in with his left wrist behind my right ear, contacting the right side of my atlas, and then rolled in with his right wrist on top of his left. Then, with his arms almost fully extended, he thrust, straightening his arms and driving that force right into my atlas. I instantly felt the warmth of circulation that went up around my skull and down my spine. I then rolled onto my back, and he re-measured my leg length. Sure enough, my half-inch-short right leg came down balanced! He re-checked my neck, and all four of those painful tender spots were gone!

When I walked out of the adjusting room, I felt a new sense of balance, a feeling like "nobody touch me; I don't want to disturb what I just got fixed." I was innately aware of the change to my body. Fortunately, it was the end of the day, so I could just go home for a good night's sleep.

When I woke up the next morning, I knew something good had happened the previous day. Recovering from my 1980 accident, I seemed to have hit an early plateau and had only gotten back a limited amount of my mental capacity. My mental retention had been severely limited since the accident, and going to school was a struggle. But it was something I wanted, so I just kept doing whatever was necessary. The day after my atlas adjustment, I had clarity. When I observed, heard, or read things, they entered a deeper level of consciousness, recording within my brain. It was like my memory banks had just gotten an upgrade from kilobytes to gigabytes.

Walking out of my trailer in Kennesaw, Georgia, that morning, I saw everything in such a vivid kaleidoscope of colors and brightness that I was forced to take notice. My next-door-neighbor's faded old yellow trailer was now the color of fresh lemons. Cotton-white clouds floated amidst a blue-sky backdrop, while to the back of my lot, trees showed off their emerald green leaves. In retrospect, I have learned that removing interference at the brain stem level improves a number of the senses, like balance, sight, and hearing.

That event sowed the seed for what would motivate me for the rest of my life. It was a personal experience so profound and life changing that I equate it to the experience of coming to know Christ as my savior.

My world had been rocked in a positive way. Although the motorcycle accident didn't fracture my skull, it definitely shifted it and my upper neck far from neutral. For that three-year lapse, I had been functioning with a misalignment. It was right under my skull: the exact location where my brain stem exits—heading south to tell my body how to function while the sensory information heads north to share what my body is sensing.

I am sure you have seen hundreds of Hollywood portrayals of what happens to the bad guy when you take his neck and twist it. Heck, even Superman in *Man of Steel*, after punching General Zod through buildings and plowing the villain through the asphalt streets, didn't even put a scratch on this bad guy from Krypton. Yet their final battle when, in the midst of blows that collapsed whole sky scrapers, the old twist-the-head move was lights out for General Zod. James Bond seems to have that move down pretty well as Agent 007; he must employ that move ten to twenty times a picture to villains worldwide.

As a chiropractor, I was a sponsor of a mixed martial arts event in Kenansville, North Carolina. Being a sponsor, I was allowed behind the scenes prior to the event, where they went over the dos and don'ts of the fight, and one "do not" makes perfect sense. You may not strike an opponent in the back of the head toward the base of the skull, though the officials allow pretty much everything else. Even mixed martial arts enthusiasts know the serious damage that can be done with a blow to this part of the body.

TAKE AWAY: WITH NEW KNOWLEDGE COMES NEW RESPONSIBILITY. IN REGARD TO THE UPPER NECK, BE IT YOURS OR YOUR LOVED ONES, SEEK OUT PROFESSIONAL CARE.

PART II

Listening to Our Bodies

Chapter Five

What Is Your Body Saying?

Most people, if they take a bold, honest look at their health picture, can tell at a glance the direction their health is going. Our bodies are equipped with an innate intelligence that often sends us pain signals as warning signs. The pain is the effect of something that is no longer in balance; something that is not working the way it was designed. The answer is not more Ibuprofen or Advil. The longer we ignore our bodies' complaints, the more dire the consequences. We turn a deaf ear to our very well-being if we don't heed our bodies' cries for help or relief. If we don't listen, no one else can.

I often use the analogy of a car. Say you run over a curb and your front end gets out of alignment. Of course, you can still drive the car, but it takes more effort to keep the car on the road. The visible change to your car is going to be lasting damage to the tires, bearings, and struts. Your options in that situation are to buy a new car, continually replace the worn out parts, or simply have the front end of your car realigned at the shop down the street. Yet, with your body the options are different. You can medicate it so that you don't hear the complaint, simply ignore it and let it get worse, or seek corrective care to get your body back in alignment. Reader, please be wise and pick the latter.

So it is, too, with the road of life we all must tread. We could choose to medicate our aching bodies in response to that slip on black ice that caused us to see white stars. We may opt to just accept the fact that we can no longer look to the left as well as to the right; our "work around" for that limited neck rotation could be to just shift our bottoms in the seat of the car when looking left. Yet, there will come a day of reckoning when your body no longer rebounds from "work arounds."

I witnessed such a day just recently in my clinic. A patient of mine, I will call her Susan, is a nurse in her forties who has already retired. She has had a lot of improvement from the care we have given her, yet she has an ongoing low-grade headache. As a nurse, Susan had sought out medical care for her aches and pains via medicine. In some cases that is the best choice; if I were to be bitten by a poisonous snake, I sure hope that someone will take me to the nearest medical clinic that can inject the necessary anti-venom into my body. Yet, for the first forty-plus years of her life, this woman has not listened correctly to what her body has been saying.

That aching low back is not due to a lack of aspirin. Susan now has a bone spur so large on her low back vertebrae that it has punctured a small hole in her spinal cord covering, allowing her cerebral spinal fluid (CSF) to leak out. That, in turn, gives her low-grade headaches. This happens because the fluid that is leaking from her low back is the same fluid that supports and surrounds her brain. Her neurologist is trying to patch up this hole in her spinal cord covering, yet so far to no avail. Hindsight being what it is, if only Susan had chosen a different answer to the prodding question of that nagging backache, she could have had a better outcome. To find the cause of the pain instead of just silencing it should be the ultimate goal; Susan should have just asked, "Why is my back hurting?" and then sought out corrective care.

Still, we were able to take Susan from debilitating headaches, which kept her bedridden for a full day every two or three weeks, to where she now has only an ongoing low-grade headache.

A medical doctor, by virtue of his profession, will give you medicine. I understand the need for medicine in cases where it is clearly applicable, such as in emergencies and with certain illnesses. However, the daily aches and pains of life are the only way our bodies can communicate with us. Deadening that language, through the use of drugs, is not always in our best interest.

God made our bodies to be self-healing, and they do a pretty good job of it. Rest, good food, exercise, and proper nervous function help our bodies travel well down the road of life. My clinic's mission statement is this: "That God would use our clinic to restore people to the way they were created to be." Bumps and bruises along the road of life happen. We need to make decisions about how we are going to respond to those injuries.

For the patients who had been dealing with "dis-ease" for years, their lists of therapies run deeply. Acupuncture is often sought as a form of therapy. Nerve blocks are an intervention that is typically attempted pretty far down the path for those seeking relief. Some of those in pain go so far as to have the nerve cauterized (surgically burned) to stop the pain signal. While there may be a bit of relief from that procedure, the nerve eventually grows back and shouts the same old message.

On X-rays, I often see disc spaces so worn that the vertebrae is bone on bone. Those patients often say, "I tried over-the-counter medication for a while. When that failed to work, I had injections into the joints of my back." The injections would work for the first one or two rounds, lasting up to six months at first. Yet they were only buying time at the expense of the body's integrity. The next step down that road is typically a surgical fusion. Had they sought out corrective care, they would have regained proper function and stability to their spinal segments.

In all our attempts to get rid of the pain, too often the main cause is not addressed. In all of life, there is always a cause and an effect. The universal law of cause and effect cannot be avoided. Suppose you ingest something that your body recognizes as potentially harmful to digest. The loose stool or the vomiting you subsequently experience is the effect. It is a reaction to a cause—in this case, what you ingested earlier. The loose stools and vomiting indicate that your body is aware of the problem and is fixing it for you, which is a healthy, normal reaction. In reference to the human body, that law plays out in many different ways but is often ignored.

If you stay up late at night to accomplish a goal and deny your body the sleep it needs, the effects of that—irritability, fatigue, and reduced function of your body's immune system—are incompatible with the vibrant life you want. The human body has certain requirements for good health that cannot be ignored. In a nutshell, these are eating a healthy diet, drinking plenty of water, exercising regularly, and sleeping well.

Sometimes the cause of an ailment can surprise us. As I am writing this, I am hindered by what is commonly called a cold. Let's take a deeper look at how this illness came about: Two days ago I was at my clinic taking X-rays for my AO work. While moving an arm of the X-ray unit, I bumped my head against the wall. I brushed it off and continued working with my new patient, hoping he didn't just see his doctor bomp his head against the wall. Later the next day, while taking care of some paperwork at the office, I started feeling ill. The typical symptoms began to creep up on me: tiredness, runny nose, sneezing, and fatigue.

While in bed that night, I noticed that my neck was sore. I had hit my head, not my neck, but there are seven vertebrae that make up the neck, which holds the skull to the body. When I struck my head that force went right to my neck, which in turn caused a shifting of those bones and thereby injured, or in medical terms "insulted," the surrounding soft tissue. That soft tissue is comprised of muscles, ligaments, and, most importantly, nerves. These nerves have jobs to do. Some of those nerves from my neck control the function of my immune system; thus, my body was overwhelmed and I became sick.

We often take our nervous system for granted. It has a lot more to do than to tell you it's hurting, yet it does that very well. The sciatica nerve is a well-known culprit that can send excruciating pain racing right through the buttocks and all the way down to the foot, even the toes in extreme cases. There are two hundred billion neurons that make up the average person's nervous system, but of that, only ten million are sensory neurons. To better picture that, say you get a slipped disk (which is a misnomer, for a disk will not slip; they will bulge or rupture and that's not good) in your low back and you irritate a nerve root the size of your thumb—Ouch! However, if you sliced your thumb-sized nerve root into twenty pieces, only one of those pieces would make you scream bloody murder.

So, what about the 95 percent of your nervous system that doesn't complain? Well, this very second the nerves in your eyes are firing off, and unless you're lying down, your postural muscles are working. If your skin is warmer than room temperature, then your heart is doing its job. And I pray the words I am sharing are being transported and stored deep in your brain by neurons as these truths sink in. You get the jest. Here is a shout-out to the silent majority, the hard-working motor nerves![2]

What this book focuses on, however, is our bodies' complaints that often go unheeded or are mistreated when a simple adjustment to the body's alignment can often provide life-changing relief. When out shopping with my wife, I often comment on fellow shoppers' gaits that are obviously altered: there should be some motion and function between the tailbone and the hip. When that dynamic function is gone, they almost seem to lurch forward with one side of their lower body. Their mobility, or lack of it, is almost painful for me to watch. Of the

---

[2] See "Difference Between Sensory and Motor Neurons," *DifferenceBetween.com*, October 25, 2013, www.differencebetween.com/difference-between-sensory-and-motor-neurons/.

ones I have questioned about it, the vast majority has been well aware of the deficit, yet few had a clue as to how to improve it, which brings me full circle back to the point of this book: Education. You don't know what you don't know. My objective is to teach a better way of dealing with that nagging headache than simply looking to what is in the medicine cabinet.

TAKE AWAY: THE WISE ONE HEARS CORRECTLY WHAT HIS BODY IS SAYING AND TAKES APPROPRIATE ACTIONS.

Chapter Six

What's with Drugs?

One patient, Dan, had tried to answer his body's complaint of severe migraines for twenty-six years with drugs. The drug cocktails he endured proved how desperately he wanted relief. Dan ended up trying a long list of drugs, with at best only a month or two of relief that would only last until his body got accustomed to what he was consuming daily. This constant need for readjustment would require him to take more medications or tweak the ones he was currently using. It doesn't take a medical degree in pharmacology to see that this is not the way to enjoy a productive, vibrant life. Relying on pharmaceuticals forces your liver to process too many different types of chemicals in the effort to stimulate or suppress your body's pain signals.[3]

Allow me to share a quote from *Killing Sacred Cows* by Garrett B. Gunderson: "We don't live by design; we live by default."[4] This is the route too many people take in reference to how they answer their bodies' complaints. I am sure readers know the answer Big Pharma has for the question "How do you spell relief?" If the answer is always R-O-L-A-I-D-S, sure it will neutralize the acid in your stomach, but let's think a little deeper.

---

[3] A good example of the ways an individual will seek change through drugs can be found in Chapter Eight with the story of Walter Payton.
[4] Garrett B. Gunderson, with Stephen Palmer, *Killing Sacred Cows: Overcoming the Financial Myths that are Destroying Your Prosperity* (Austin, TX: Greenleaf Book Group, 2008), 235.

Why is there acid in your stomach? Could it be that it is part of the natural process of how our bodies break food down into the nutrients that sustain us? If we keep diluting the acid levels in our stomachs, then the food we eat won't be properly processed when it travels down the rest of our digestive tract. That, in turn, could cause problems on two fronts: our bodies will not be able to absorb the nutrients if the food is not broken down properly, and further down the intestinal tract has to work harder to deal with partially digested food due to the lack of acid.

Throughout the digestive tract, there are key spots where certain minerals and vitamins are absorbed and utilized. A good example is Vitamin B-6. Some people need B-6 injections, not because the vitamin is not present in their diets but because the receptor sites in the small intestines cannot pick the nutrient up due to irritation of that lining, which prevents vitamin absorption. If Rolaids or another form of antacid were to become a person's standard form of relief, then something else is going on inside his or her body, and the antacid is only masking the symptoms of greater, unresolved problems.

Another slogan comes to mind, this one for Chiffon Margarine: "It's not nice to fool Mother Nature." When we think we can do better than our Creator, we need to think again. In margarine, the chemical nature is altered and our bodies cannot process that variation at the molecular level. The nutritional value of margarine has been debated for years; it's even been said to be one molecular change short of becoming plastic! So, too, is there a debate about the habitual use of Advil, Tylenol, and many other common drugs.

Individuals who have lived on Nonsteroidal Anti-inflammatory Drugs (NSAIDs) have two issues to deal with. First, the joints of their bodies, which have been howling at their owners long enough to develop a habit of taking NSAIDs, will begin to break down due to the ongoing irritation not being resolved. That is when arthritis begins to set up shop. Second, the manufacturers of NSAIDs have gathered enough data on the effects of their product on the liver that they now report that acetaminophen will, if too much is taken, damage the liver. Professional athletes have long relied on NSAIDs, although more and more athletes are adding chiropractors to their teams.[5]

Many of you may recall that old jingle, "Plop! Plop! Fizz! Fizz! Oh, what a relief it is!" I'm in my fifties, and I remember that jingle from my childhood. In the midst of writing this book, I discovered the following caution on the back of an Alka-Seltzer Plus product:

Liver warning: This product contains acetaminophen. Severe liver damage may occur if you take

- more than 8 tablets in 24 hours, which is the maximum daily amount for this product
- with other drugs containing acetaminophen
- three or more alcoholic drinks every day while using this product.

I would surmise that they were required to put that warning on their products because research has proved the risk of liver damage. Undoubtedly, similar warnings can be found on a host of products on the drug store shelves. According to the website KnowYourDose.org, "Acetaminophen is the most common drug ingredient in America. There are more than 600 medicines which contain acetaminophen, including over-the-counter (OTC) and prescription (Rx) medicines."[6]

The medical profession and pharmaceutical industry have come a long way in finding ways to block what the body is saying, and they have gotten pretty good at it. Yet, is it wiser to

---

[5] See Chapter Eight, "Chiropractic and Sports."
[6] "Common Medicines," *KnowYourDose.org*, www.knowyourdose.org/common-medicines/.

deaden the noise of an aching joint or resolve the cause of the symptoms? The latter, I think, is God's intention because He built us with a nervous system that can sense when something is not right. Let's return to my analogy of the car: Is it better to have your car's front-end alignment straightened out or to drive your car down the road of life until the wheels fall off?

If you are going through life trying to dumb down what your body is trying to tell you, stop and think. I often use this analogy: How long do you need to hold your hand on a hot burner before taking action? Do you need to smell the malodor of burning flesh to know you need to react to the pain signal? Your body is talking to you, are you going to listen or simply tell it to be quiet? When you go to a dentist with a toothache, you wouldn't simply want him to make the pain go away. You would want to find out why it's hurting, what's wrong and fix the problem.

One of my soul (spelling intentional) purposes in writing this book is to share the knowledge I have learned, first as a patient who has been through it and now as a chiropractor providing care for others. People don't know what they don't know. Chiropractic doctors serve less than 10 percent of the US population because the therapy we offer can't compete with Big Pharma, which runs untold numbers of advertisements and commercials costing millions of dollars each year. We, as chiropractors, try to show one patient at a time that there is a better way to live. In Latin, the word *doctor* means *teacher*, and it behooves us, as chiropractors, to educate patients. If people's education is limited to what radio and television tells them, they'll only know to apply the remedies those thousands of commercials advertise instead of getting themselves back into alignment and optimal health.

TAKE AWAY: IN REGARD TO YOUR HEALTH CARE OPTIONS, CONSUMERS BEWARE.

PART III

The Importance of Alignment to Well-Being

Chapter Seven

A History of Chiropractic

According to the book *Chiropractic First* by Terry A. Rondberg, DC,[7] the earliest records of spinal manipulation can be found in cave drawings in Point le Merd in southwestern France. These drawings are believed to date back to 17500 BC. Records of the practice of spinal manipulation in China date back to 2700 BC. The ancient Greeks solved low-back problems by maneuvering the legs. Historical records show ancient Egyptians knew the health benefits of straight spines, and the "ancient Japanese, Egyptians, Babylonians, Hindus, Tibetans, and Syrians practiced spinal manipulative therapy."[8]

In 300 BC, Hippocrates, the Father of Medicine, said, "Look well to the spine for the cause of disease."[9] At about the same time, Herodotus was curing diseases by correcting spinal abnormalities through exercise. If the patient was too weak to exercise, Herodotus manipulated their spines. Philosopher Aristotle did not approve of Herodotus's work because, as he put it, "he made old men young and thus prolonged their lives too greatly," at a time when the average lifespan was about thirty years.[10]

---

[7] Terry A. Rondberg, *Chiropractic First: The Fastest Growing Healthcare Choice . . . Before Drugs or Surgery* (Chiropractic Journal, 1998).
[8] Ibid., 8.
[9] Ibid.
[10] Ibid., 9.

The Greeks created machines to stretch the spine and correct dislocations. They also hung patients by their heels or walked on their backs to correct spinal problems. By 200 AD, physician Claudius Galen was teaching proper positions and relations in the spinal column. He was called the Prince of Physicians after healing the paralyzed right hand of a scholar simply by aligning the man's neck vertebrae.

Fast forward several hundred years to Iowa, where Daniel David (D.D.) Palmer raised bees, sold sweet raspberries, and taught school before becoming interested in magnetic healing in 1885. Magnetic healing—an alternative medical practice that involves the use of static magnetic fields—was a common therapy at the time, which used the body's magnetic properties. In 1887 D.D. Palmer moved his family to Davenport, Iowa, where he opened the Palmer Cure & Infirmary. It was there, in 1895, that D.D. Palmer made his first chiropractic adjustment. The procedure was performed on janitor Harvey Lillard, who had been deaf for seventeen years. As D.D. Palmer described it:

> Harvey Lillard...could not hear the racket of a wagon on the street or the ticking of a watch. I made inquiry as to the cause of his deafness and was informed that when he was exerting himself in a cramped, stooping position, he felt something give way in his back and immediately became deaf.
>
> An examination showed a vertebra racked from its normal position. I reasoned that if that vertebra was replaced, the man's hearing should be restored. With this object in view, a half hour's talk persuaded Mr. Lillard to allow me to replace it. I racked it into position by using the spinous process as a lever, and soon the man could hear as before.
>
> There was nothing accidental about this as it was accomplished with an object in view, and the result expected was

obtained. There was nothing 'crude' about this adjustment; it was specific, so much so that no other Chiropractor has equaled it.[11]

While Palmer knew what to do and how to do it, he was puz-
zled as to why his methods worked. He treated heart problems,
epilepsy, stomach disorders, chronic pain, poor vision, and
many other health problems by making adjustments to patients'
spines so that their bodies functioned normally. Palmer coined
the term *chiropractic* from the Greek *chiro*, meaning hands,
and *practice*, meaning practice or operation.

Despite its success in treating a host of maladies, the emerg-
ing modern practice of chiropractic therapy did have its detrac-
tors. In 1905 Palmer was arrested for practicing medicine
without a license, although he had used neither surgery nor
drugs on his patients. He was sentenced to one hundred and
five days in jail and fined $350.[12] Chiropractic started out as a
"social and political phenomenon in the early part of the last
century," but "not everyone was happy with its popularity."[13] In
his book *Old School Wisdom*, Dr. Jeffry Finnigan, writing as Dr.
Finn, tells of other chiropractors who were jailed for practicing
medicine without licenses despite the fact that they, too, admin-
istered no drugs nor did they perform any surgeries.

In 1918, during the flu pandemic, people experienced
remarkable benefits under chiropractic care. Put simply, the
structure of the spine influences the function on the nervous system, especially the sympathetic nervous system, which controls

---

[11] Ibid., 12.

[12] Using the David Manuel.com Inflation Calculator, $350 in 1905 equals $9,467.46
in 2016.

[13] Jeffry Finnigan (writing as Dr. Finn), *Old School Wisdom for Longevity and Pain
Free Living* (Bend, OR: Jeffry Finnigan, DC, BCAO, 2015), 41.

and regulates the immune system.[14] Some were neither swayed nor thrilled by the discipline's achievements. During the first half of the twentieth century, the medical profession was at war with chiropractic. Finn states:

> By 1901, all of the United States had given the medical profession authority to set standards and police itself. That "authority" then used the courts to turn on and prosecute chiropractors. They lobbied state legislatures to block licensing the profession of chiropractic. In 1905 D.D. Palmer was one of the first to be convicted and jailed for practicing chiropractic. It is estimated that, by 1931, 12,000 chiropractors had undergone 15,000 prosecutions for practicing medicine without a license![15]

Crowds of up to twelve hundred patients protested these arrests. Patients did not want to testify against their doctors and were subsequently "subpoenaed and treated as hostile witnesses."[16]

> Some of the prosecuted chiropractors would pay a fine and simply return to practice later that afternoon, facing further prosecutions. For this reason, some chiropractors would choose jail time over fines. These were not the jails of today—they would have rats and bugs and could include hard labor. More than 100,000 letters were sent to the prison where a husband and wife chiropractic team was sent for one hundred days.[17]

Some imprisoned chiropractors practiced their art while behind bars, even treating patients who came to the jails for help.

[14] Dr. Dan Murphy, comments at a Coast Chiropractic Kawana seminar, February 6, 2017.
[15] Finnigan, *Old School Wisdom*, 41.
[16] Ibid.
[17] Ibid., 42.

According to Finnigan, "Arrests of chiropractors in the United States continued from 1906 until 1974, when Louisiana became the fiftieth state to license chiropractors."[18] Nevertheless, as Dr. Roy Sweat pointed out in reference to chiropractic as well as to life in general, "If it's right, it will come out on the top. If it's wrong, given time, regardless of who is trying to prop something up, it will fail."[19]

As for D.D. Palmer, he died of typhoid fever at the age of sixty-eight in 1913. Along with the art of chiropractic, Palmer left his son, Bartlett Joshua Palmer (or B.J., as he was known) to continue his work. Although the two often argued and went their separate ways over such issues as the use of X-rays (D.D. was against and B.J. was in favor), it was B.J. who would further develop the practice his father had discovered.

TAKE AWAY: ANCIENT AND MODERN PEOPLE ALIKE HAVE OBSERVED THIS TRUTH: GOD DOESN'T MAKE JUNK; HE HAS A DESIRED POSITION FOR EACH BONE IN YOUR BODY AND ANY DEVIATION FROM THAT IS NOT GOING TO BE FOR THE BETTER.

---

[18] Ibid., 44.
[19] Quoted in Finnigan, *Old School Wisdom*, 44.

Chapter Eight

Chiropractic and Sports

Professional athletes are a strong and influential bunch. Known for outrageous lifestyles and salaries, they seem to be overcompensated, golden icons. But the sad fact is that many of these men and women live with unbearable pain every day of their lives.

Professional athletes spend most of their lives training in their chosen sports. Many of these athletes start at a young age. Together, this means a lot of time is spent pushing their bodies to the extremes needed to succeed in professional sports. In doing this, they have a greater chance of going too far and injuring themselves. In particular, a great number of professional athletes, depending on their chosen sport, can and do endure a lot of trauma to their heads and necks. For anyone who has watched football, it's obvious that these guys are hurting their bodies. Blows that send helmets sailing are not good for anyone's noggin. Football, soccer, rugby, and hockey...the list of injury-prone sports goes on and on. Those blows to the body and skull can take their toll. This is all the more true the younger the athlete was when he or she began playing.

An example of a sports injury in a young athlete is given by one of my patients, Noah. He came to me for relief after sustaining a football injury at the age of fourteen. Noah said his headaches "would get so bad that I couldn't do anything because of the pain." He could not pay attention in his classes, for the headaches were so bad that he had to lie down, close his eyes, and try not to engage his brain. It was so painful, that, for half a year, Noah didn't even go to school. For a player who was once active on a junior varsity football team, it was quite a blow to not even be able to run due to the pain in his head. The injury definitely altered the normal activity of this otherwise healthy fourteen-year-old boy.

After just two treatments to realign the bones in Noah's neck, he wrote the following testimonial:

> May 20, 2016
>
> Before the treatment, I was hit on the top of the head in football, pressing my head straight down. I had a headache since September 2015 and started seeing Patrick [Gallagher] on May 13, 2016. The headache would spike periodically. It would get so bad that I couldn't do anything because of the pain. I tried about everything. I went to Duke Hospital, East Carolina University, and a [different] chiropractor. I took so much meds they gave me stomach pains. A friend recommended [atlas] orthogonal chiropractic because it helped her, so I tried it and right after he [Dr. Gallagher] moved my atlas my headache basically disappeared. I think this is the only thing that worked to relieve my headaches.

Fortunately for Noah, he discovered a path to recovery that was both natural and effective: atlas orthogonal chiropractic. But many athletes are not so lucky. The cases of pro football players Jerry Rice and Walter Payton are good comparisons of the difference in outcomes between treating such injuries with chiropractic care verses drugs. Rice used chiropractic therapy and Payton took the other route.

National Football League (NFL) wide receiver Jerry Rice played twenty seasons in the NFL from 1985 to 2004. His first fifteen years were with the San Francisco 49ers, followed by three years playing for the Oakland Raiders, with his final year as a Seattle Seahawk. He believes so strongly in the value of chiropractic care that he posted a video tribute to chiropractors on YouTube.[20] While the average playing career for an NFL athlete is only three and a half years,[21] in his testimony Rice credits his ability to play professional football for twenty seasons to the chiropractors who kept him in the game, proving that this player was getting something extra to keep him up and running.

Rice remembers taking hits from players he describes as "nearly twice my size" (he weighed in at more than two hundred pounds) and admits suffering repeated injuries. His first visit to a chiropractor happened shortly before his team, the San Francisco 49ers, played the Cincinnati Bengals in Super Bowl XXIII in 1989. "A couple of our players were injured and a chiropractor turned things around," Rice recalls.[22] Deciding he had nothing to lose, Rice was treated by a chiropractor. He went on to make an 85-yard touchdown catch, winning the Super Bowl for his team.

After retiring from football, Rice competed on the popular television program *Dancing with the Stars*. He recounts the challenges and exhaustion of the show, saying it was "not as brutal" as football but that it gave him a new perspective on aches and pains. Rice used the help of chiropractors to stay competitive during the filming.

"I believe in you," Rice said, addressing the chiropractors who view his video.

Now retired from both football and dancing, Rice says he still uses chiropractors to keep him healthy and active in the

---

[20] "Jerry Rice Speaks on the Value of Chiropractic Care," *YouTube*, August 5, 2011, www.youtube.com/watch?v=YWoiiKy4xGs.
[21] Jeff Nelson, "The Longest Professional Sports Careers," *RSVLTS*, July 23, 2013, *www.rsvlts.com/2013/07/22/longest-sports-careers.*
[22] "Jerry Rice Speaks."

game of life. He says chiropractic gives him the edge he needs to live his life to the fullest. "You help millions," Rice says in the video. He is a spokesman for the Foundation for Chiropractic Progress (F4CP), reaching out to millions of people about the cause and educating the public about the importance of chiropractic care.

Now comes the story of a professional football player with a different outcome, as told in the biography *Sweetness: The Enigmatic Life of Walter Payton* by Jeff Pearlman.[23]

According to Pearlman, the Chicago Bears player and Hall of Famer was "suicidal, abusing pain medication and dealing with a crumbling family situation" by the mid-1990s.[24] Payton had played thirteen seasons for the NFL, retiring in 1987. At that time, he held the record as the leading rusher in NFL history. Payton's agent, Bud Holmes, received calls from Payton in which the athlete spoke of wanting to take his own life.[25] For all his greatness and celebrity, Payton was feeling lonely and unloved.

Like most professional athletes, Payton had accrued a lot of pain and injury. He used pills and elixirs, including a "cocktail of Tylenol and Vicodin," to deal with the pain, according to Holmes.[26] "Walter was pounding his body with medication," Holmes said. "I wish I knew how bad it was, but at the time I really didn't."[27] In 1988, Payton visited several dental offices complaining of tooth pain, securing several prescriptions for morphine. At least one pharmacist was concerned and called

[23] Jeff Pearlman, *Sweetness: The Enigmatic Life of Walter Payton* (New York: Gotham Books, 2011).
[24] "Book Describes Troubled Walter Payton," *ESPN.com*, September 29, 2011, www.espn.com/chicago/nfl/story/_/id/7031006/chicago-bears-walter-payton-used-drugs-talked-suicide-according-book.
[25] Ibid.
[26] Ibid.
[27] Ibid.

the police, but, perhaps due to his celebrity status, Payton only received a warning from the officers who visited him. The grim reality was that he also had a tank of nitrous oxide in his garage to combat the problems he faced.[28]

Payton was inducted into the Pro Football Hall of Fame in 1993, a day that should have been purely joyful but was instead very tense, as both his wife, Connie, and his mistress arrived for the ceremonies, an example of how confused even his home life had become. The two women were kept from seeing one another by Cindy Quirk, Payton's assistant, who recalled their presence as "ships passing in the night." She later added, "I can't describe the horror of that trip."[29] The Paytons were separated at the time but had not gone public with that information in order to protect their children and Walter's reputation. Later, Connie Payton would have a meeting with the mistress, telling her, "You can have him. He doesn't want me or the children."[30]

Due to drug abuse, Payton died of a rare liver disease, primary sclerosing cholangitis (PSC),[31] and bile duct cancer in November 1999 at the age of 45.

The liver filters everything. Too much medication—prescription, over-the-counter, or other—causes liver damage. With too many drugs in Payton's body, a toxic environment was created, taxing his liver as it worked to filter out all those chemicals. The byproduct of this additional stress was liver failure. (As I write this, a member of my local church was admitted to the University of North Carolina Medical Center at

---

[28] Ibid.
[29] Ibid.
[30] Ibid.
[31] The American Liver Foundation defines primary sclerosing cholangitis (PSC) as a chronic disease that slowly damages the bile ducts, causing bile to accumulate in the liver and promoting the development of cirrhosis or fibrosis of the liver. PSC may also lead to bile duct cancer. "Primary Sclerosing Cholangitis (PSC)," *American Liver Foundation*, www.liverfoundation.org/abouttheliver/info/psc/.

Chapel Hill for a similar liver problem. Our friend had never used illegal drugs and was not a drinker but had endured many years of antibiotic and NSAID use.) How much simpler would it have been for Payton, and countless others like him, to have his spine analyzed to find the cause of "dis-ease" instead of masking symptoms with powerful drugs, to step back and see the bigger picture of what was really going on?

Teams want their players to be healthy. A modern NFL health care team would not use the "no pain, no gain" treatment principles depicted in the 1979 motion picture *North Dallas Forty*. Scenes in that movie showed players receiving multiple shots of anesthetics for torn ligaments and tendons so that they could continue playing. Their bodies were saying, "Wait a second, I need some time to heal here."

Dr. Sol Cogan, who worked on the sidelines for the Detroit Lions from 2002 to 2015, says athletes, their agents, athletic trainers, and medical doctors understand the consequences of disabling the pain mechanism. These health professionals have come to align themselves with the chiropractic perspective: treat the cause of the pain. In fact, there's even a Professional Football Chiropractic Society (PFCS) that seeks to discover and share best practices among each other and with chiropractors who work with other pro sports teams. Of course, chiropractic care doesn't have to be reserved only for professional athletes; amateur athletes could and should experience the benefits of proper body alignment as well.

Turning to a sport played by many just for fun, we see how chiropractic care keeps golfers on the greens. Chiropractor Michael Dorausch explains: "There are three fundamental causes of golf injuries: poor posture, lack of flexibility, and poor swing mechanics. The root cause of poor mechanics is often a result of a physical restriction or mechanical dysfunction, which may be alleviated through chiropractic procedures. Lack of flexibility can also be addressed by treatment and a prescribed stretching program specifically designed around each patient's restrictions. Obviously, chiropractic care is ideally suited to deal with poor posture."[32]

"Lifting weights and seeing a chiropractor on a regular basis has made me a better golfer," said golf legend Tiger Woods. "I've been going to chiropractors for as long as I can remember. It is as important to my training as practicing my swing."[33] Woods even rode on the Chiropractic Centennial float in the 1995 Pasadena Tournament of Roses Parade, whose theme for the year was Sports—A Quest for Excellence. At the time, Woods was only nineteen years old and chiropractic was turning one hundred. His achievements at that time included becoming the ninth player to win consecutive US amateur championships, being voted Pac-10 player of the year, becoming an NCAA first-team All-American, being awarded Stanford's Male Freshman of the Year, and participating in his first PGA major tournament. In 1997, at age twenty-one, Tiger Woods was the leading money winner on the PGA tour, with a record $2,066,833 in earnings. He won the Masters, his first major championship, by the widest margin of victory the tournament had ever seen (twelve strokes) and became the youngest Masters winner ever. He also won three other PGA events that year. Throughout that great year in Tiger Woods's career, he was kept in alignment by his chiropractor, Dr. Jeff Spencer.

Dr. Armen Manoucherian, from Glendale, California, wrote:

> In order to hit a golf ball well and consistently, your body must be balanced. In addition, many injuries associated

[32] Michael Dorausch, "Tiger Woods Wins British Open: A Chiropractic Story," *Planet Chiropractic*, July 25, 2006, www.planetc1.com/search/tiger-woods-wins-british-open-a-chiropractic-story.html.
[33] Armen Manoucherian, "Why Does Tiger Woods Regularly See a Chiropractor?" *Health Edge*, November 20, 2013, http://healthedgela.com/why-does-tiger-woods-regularly-see-a-chiropractor.

with golfing such as back, hip, knee, ankle, and neck injuries can frequently be prevented if you are regularly keeping your spine in proper alignment. During the first leg of
the 2013 FedEx cup golf playoffs, Tiger was struggling with
back spasms after sleeping on a particularly uncomfortable mattress. Even with back spasms, he was able to come
within one shot of forcing a playoff. This type of physical resiliency is common with chiropractic patients. With
a properly functioning spine and nervous system you are
able to adapt with injuries and stresses more effectively.
In a nutshell: Life "in" alignment = "advantage" on the golf
course, while life "out" of alignment = "disadvantage."[34]

Manoucherian continued, "Chiropractic care is focused on
keeping the spine and nervous system balanced and working
optimally. Misalignments in the spinal column lead to muscle
imbalances, postural changes, unequal weight distribution and
slower reaction times."[35]

Casual athletes and amateurs cannot typically withstand the
rigors and the intensity that great sports champions endure.
There are enormous emotional and physical demands involved
for professional players. Their training requires concentration,
self-discipline, and mental toughness. It is easy to discuss these
qualities and characteristics but quite difficult to emulate them.
Perseverance, focus, and emotion are all qualities of champions. At 122 years old this year, the chiropractic profession is
widely recognized as one such champion, not only as a form of
natural health care for the world's greatest athletes but also as
the leading form of natural health care for the people that love
them, cheer for them, and strive to be like them.

---

[34] Ibid.
[35] Ibid.

Whether you're paid millions or simply love the sport, we're all athletes. Everybody needs to get and keep their heads on straight to play their very best.

TAKE AWAY: TO TRULY SEE HOW WELL YOU CAN PERFORM AS AN ATHLETE, IT BEHOOVES YOU TO MAKE SURE YOU'RE IN ALIGNMENT.

Chapter Nine

Performing Well in Alignment

Whether or not you are an athlete, proper alignment supports optimal functioning and well-being. The following testimonial is from a mother who is very involved in the lives of her athletic kids as well as being a runner herself.

> Dr. Gallagher is amazing. Not only is he filled with knowledge and competency in his field, he has a wonderful "bedside manner." Not only have I gained considerable relief from various pain throughout my body (back, hips, neck, elbows, fingers) but Dr. Gallagher has given me advice about proper body alignment for walking/running. This knowledge, in turn, allows me to exercise without pain. I would highly recommend Chiropractic First [Dr. Gallagher's clinic] without hesitation, and in fact, have done so.

Another sports-related testimonial comes from one of my teenaged patients. Mitch was a treat to treat. He came to my office on a referral from his grandparents, who had responded quite favorably to the care I had provided for them.

> Dear Dr. Gallagher:
> Thank you for accepting me as one of your patients. Through God and your help, I no longer play with pain in baseball at Wayne County Day School. Before coming to you I was in constant pain especially with my arm.

My elbow prevented me from pitching. The most I could throw would be about two innings in relief. Since coming to you I have been able to pitch a complete game without difficulty. As you can see from the *Goldsboro News Argus* article, my pitching has made a complete turnaround. I give you the credit and God the Glory for this miraculous recovery. Thank you, Dr. Gallagher.

Sincerely,

Mitch Turnage

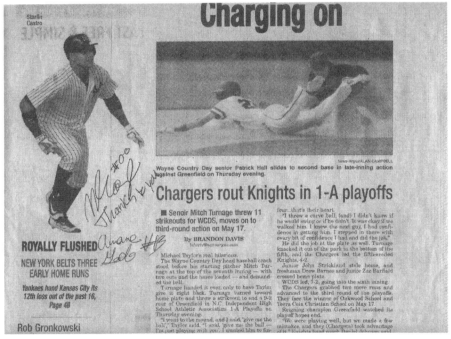

Mitch's winning performance, where he pitched the whole game and struck out eleven batters.

Mitch came in with a specific problem: pitching caused pain! Although his elbow was in pain, it was actually his shoulder blade that was the problem; it was being displaced by the speed of his pitch due to the underdeveloped muscles holding his shoulder to his body. As we adjusted his shoulder, his pitching improved, proving once again the importance of alignment. After that, my reputation spread throughout the school, which allowed me to teach the cross-country track team there about a better form for running with Chi Running. My first season assisting the team, the girls won the North Carolina state finals in 1-A High School Cross-Country Track.

With a natural love of running myself, I have been blessed to have a profound understanding of how the body functions. As I combined my interest with knowledge from my field, I was impressed with the outcome. Eventually, I learned the secret to marathon running. Not surprisingly, it involves proper alignment.

I started running marathons in 2005. Unbeknownst to me, I was damaging my body. Like many people, I assumed that you just trained to run and then ran the race. Of course, there is an awful lot of training if you want to run 26.2 miles at one time, but I thought, as Nike says, "Just do it." It was during my training runs of twenty-plus miles that the physical toll began to mount on my frame. There I was, a chiropractor seeing two other chiropractors yet failing to improve my low-back pain. My back hurt so much that I could not even raise my arms in church. Fortunately, my wife saw an advertisement for a running class in Chapel Hill, North Carolina, called Chi Running.

At the class, I relearned how to run. A focus on the slant of my body, foot strike, cadence, muscle usage, and more came into play when I truly began to run correctly. Putting to work what Danny Dreyer, the inventor of Chi Running, taught began to make an impact not only in my ability to run without hurting myself but also in my body: I now could run pain free.[36] Taking Dreyer's class gave me a better comprehension of the importance of alignment in running. I began engaging my core

---

[36] See Appendix A for a guide to performing Chi Stretch.

strength, thus allowing for proper pelvic leveling. As I engaged my core muscles, my pelvis leveled off and I found that I could hold my body in a better position. Once in this proper form, my body was well balanced and grounded. As the Chinese say, when you are not engaging your core muscles to correct your form, you are spilling your Chi—your life force—through your bad posture. This is referred to as slouching, where your pelvis drops in the front, causing your shoulders to roll forward. Posture is how you balance your body. When your shoulders roll forward, your mid-back, between your shoulder blades, arches backward, creating a hunchback. This is made all the more pronounced when you place your head way forward, in a position called "anterior carriage." All this happens when your foundation is dropped and you default to slouching.

Naturally, if you have all of those postural distortions going on in addition to a deviated atlas that is putting your head off-center, you're headed into troubled waters. Plainly and simply, God didn't create you to go through life that way. The added stress and strain to simple daily activities will leave you way short of optimal living. The seeming increase in the number of joint replacements isn't solely due to the fact that we are living longer but to the fact that we are living "crooked lives." This pelvic imbalance, which could be secondary to a crooked head, creates femoral socket degeneration, not to mention degenerative disc diseases of the lumbar spine, which cause sciatica; dropped foot, which is where the nerve to your foot is irritated due to a nerve blockage; and common low-back pain.

I have seen the effects of poor posture time and time again in my clinic. It is something I go over on X-rays when I point out a leg-length discrepancy. I ask my patients, "Which way does weight go, uphill or downhill?" The majority gets this right and say, "Downhill." I then show them their hip-height difference. If it is larger than five millimeters, after a few years the spacing around the ball and socket of the lower hip will become smaller. The bone above the leg on that side will become denser due to the added stress. A very common occurrence in degenerative disc disease is that bone spurs develop as the vertebrae approach each other due to the stress of this imbalance.

Muscle spasms, for instance, are a common warning that joints have gone beyond their limit. When muscles spasm it is a sign that the body is trying to deal with an injured or unstable segment. I see that in the clinic with patients who have low-back pain. This usually indicates that they have had some slippage of the vertebral segments of their low back, and their bodies are trying to stabilize it. Yet Big Pharma says, "Simply take a muscle relaxer and you'll be fine. Of course it is going to be painful too, and we gotcha covered there with a pain pill that will make you forget you even have a back." But once you ingest that muscle relaxer, it affects your whole body. What is the downside of that? It's twofold: First, it silences the segment of your body that is asking for support and stability—the body's message just got trumped by that medication. Second, think of the most important muscle in your body. Hint: you put your hand over this every time you say the Pledge of Allegiance. Your heart already has a tough job as it pumps blood through more than 60,000 miles of blood vessels throughout your body three times every minute! Do you really want to tell that muscle to relax?

I see a number of my patients, at varying ages, find a new alignment to live from, meaning that whatever activities are expected at their age, as long as they maintain their corrections, they should be able to do them. Be that running a marathon, climbing a mountain, playing a round of eighteen holes of golf, or picking up a grandchild, if their bodies are in proper alignment these things are doable. Inversely, though, if your body is not performing at the same level as that of your peers, as I said in Chapter Five, your body is talking to you, and you had better listen.

TAKE AWAY: TAKE IT FROM ME, THERE IS A RIGHT WAY AND A WRONG WAY TO RUN A MARATHON, INCLUDING THE MARATHON THAT IS OUR DAILY LIVES.

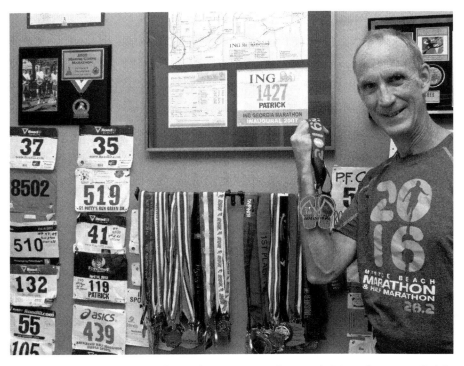

The medal I'm holding is from the 2016 Myrtle Beach Marathon. My finish time was three hours and thirty-eight minutes. If I can take eight minutes off my time I could qualify for the Boston Marathon, which is my goal.

Photo Credit: Calvin N. Sanders, C&B Photography LLC

PART IV

The Importance of Head Alignment and the Benefits of Atlas Orthogonal Care

Chapter Ten

Neuroanatomy 101

So far we've discussed why it is important to listen to the pain signals your body is sending you and how proper bodily alignment supports optimal functioning. But, did you know that there are many unfortunate individuals who go through life with their heads on crooked? In this section, you'll discover a very important bone in the spinal column, the atlas, and will learn about the myriad ways it can affect total body function if it is misaligned. You'll also be introduced to a little-known specialty, atlas orthogonal chiropractic, which has made tremendous changes in the lives of patients by making small, delicate adjustments by compressional energy wave for the correction of a misaligned atlas.

Place the beds of your thumbnails together with one thumb pad facing up and the other facing down. This represents what is called a lateral mass of the atlas. As a miniature model of the anatomy of the neck, one thumb pad makes contact with "the skull" while the other makes contact with "the axis," the second bone in the neck. The atlas is essentially a ring of bone surrounding the brain stem that rests on top of the axis, but bear in mind that you have two thumb-size masses to support the skull that lie just outside the hole in the bottom of your skull where the brain stem exits. The brain stem is an important part of your neuroanatomy. This all-important extension of your brain lies within millimeters of the most mobile and lightest segment of your spine, the atlas, which solely supports your skull. Being so

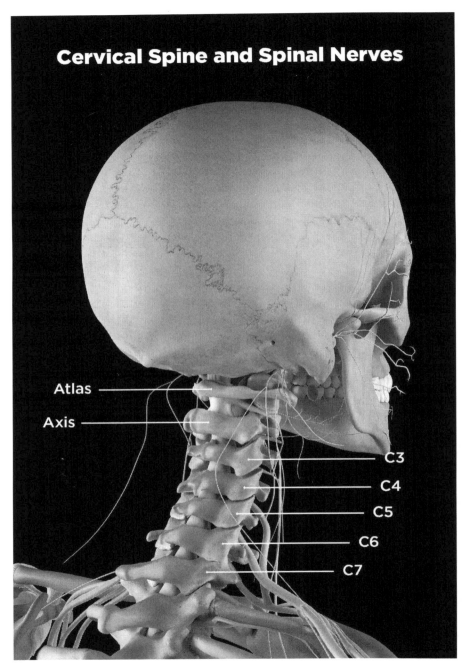

Photo Credit: sciencerf ©123RF.com

close to the brain stem, a minute misalignment in the atlas can have a huge impact. The atlas has to be light for mobility. It has to rock and rotate as we nod and turn our heads. By contrast, the axis has to be much larger to deal with the stress of supporting the weight of the skull. To locate the atlas, take your right hand and feel just below the bottom of your right ear, you will find a small knob of bone extending from your skull downward, this is called the mastoid process. Moving just one fingertip down and forward from that tip will place your finger right on top of the transverse process, the outside part of your own atlas!

The *medulla oblongata* is the brain stem. Essentially all the neurological information leaving and returning to the skull, shy the twelve cranial nerves, travels via the brain stem and through the *foramen magnum*, which is Greek for "large opening." This opening is located at the base of the skull. What happens here is the key part of my work and the results we get! The atlas is located at this highly critical neurological area. The brain stem is centered within that highly mobile and ever so light atlas vertebrae. That's why any deviations here can and do cause a lot of major neurological problems. My aim is to remove that deviation.

Once I became involved with performing AO work, I noticed a pattern I termed the "Mad Mommy Syndrome." The name is an allusion to the old adage "If Mama ain't happy, ain't nobody happy," and I enjoy explaining this to my patients because as they come to understand this phenomenon it adds to their understanding of the importance of the atlas work I do. In addition to adjusting the atlas, I use another chiropractic technique called Activator to adjust the other twenty-three spinal segments in addition to the extremities. Yet, when a patient's atlas is out of alignment, I often mention that they have the Mad Mommy Syndrome, meaning that the insult located at the top of the spine is, in a sense, so loud that I can't ascertain what else is going on south of the atlas. The neurological insult at the brain stem is so disturbing to the patient's body that I have a hard time getting an accurate reading on where the rest of the problem truly lies. That is why it is important to make sure the atlas is corrected first, getting the patient's head back on straight so that the doctor can clearly see what else needs to be corrected.

If the atlas is out of alignment and the nervous system is irritated at the brain stem level, you're not going to be a "happy camper." I once had a family of three generations under my care for a number of years, and all were well educated on the importance of the atlas work I was doing. One visit the husband said to me, "I think my wife's atlas is out. She is such a b**** today." I saw his wife later that week and, sure enough, her atlas had shifted to the left of her skull and twisted forward. I adjusted her atlas and apparently her disposition because those in her life noticed how she was at ease that evening. It's hard to be the loving wife, helpful husband, concerned parent, or even just a decent person when your body is not at ease. One doesn't need to be a neurophysiologist to know that an insult to this level of your nervous system will, at the very least, prevent you from being good company.

Often, however, atlas misalignment and the resulting insults to the nervous system manifest in far more serious ways. The brain requires more blood than any other organ of the body. If someone had a serious scalp wound, you would see lots of blood flowing. Think about it: when you get up too fast and you get dizzy, what has just happened? Exactly: the blood supply to your brain just went south, and your body is telling you so in no uncertain terms. In a worst-case scenario, the dizziness will cause you to fall to the ground, putting your brain at the same level as your heart so that the blood flow to the brain is level, no longer fighting an uphill battle. This is one reason it is so important to get people who are in a state of shock to lie down and elevate their feet; it puts less stress on the brain.

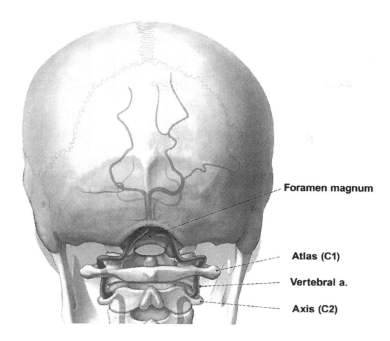

Image credit: RW Sweat Foundation

The term *atlas neurovascular syndrome* (ANVS) points out the two main effects when the atlas is subluxated, or out of joint: one is vascular and the other is neurological. The vascular effect is similar to putting a kink in a garden hose. The midbrain, which plays a role in vision, hearing, motor control, sleep, alertness, and temperature regulation, gets 80 percent of its blood supply from one artery, called the vertebral artery. This artery travels through the bone you placed your finger on at the beginning of this chapter. As it travels through the transverse process, the vertebral artery makes four sharp turns in a very short distance. When the atlas misaligns, or subluxates, not only does it go to the side of your skull but it also rotates forward or backward. Traveling up the neck, at the atlas location, that important artery first goes away from the body, then up through the atlas, then back toward the body before finally bending north to go into the brain. All those turns happen in a short space. Now imagine the atlas twisting, which it will do when it is subluxated, or misaligned, and you can get a glimpse of the importance of proper atlas alignment: any disturbance in that blood vessel can be critical.

Due to that restriction of blood at the brain stem level from an atlas misalignment, I have had patients with extreme vertigo. Some even have to walk down the clinic hallway holding onto the wall for balance. After I adjust their atlases, removing the rotation and freeing up the blood flow to their brains, they are able to stand upright and walk straight again. In most cases, the amount of restriction caused by the atlas rotation directly relates to the severity of their symptoms.

The typical patient would seek out an atlas orthogonalist for the "neuro" side of ANVS. Take my wife, Blondine, for example. She had bad migraines before we met; they had developed in her teenage years. These migraines were caused by misalignments in her neck, more specifically in her upper neck. The misalignment was evident when viewing Blondine's cervical X-rays. In reviewing her X-rays with a colleague, Dr. Bill Macchi, also a Board Certified Atlas Orthogonal (BCAO) chiropractor, I pointed out the deviations. I said, in Blondine's presence, "With the shape of that neck, I think this patient ought to marry a chiropractor." Blondine had a big smile on her face, for I had already "gotten on my knee" a month earlier. With a few adjustments, her headaches cleared up and she didn't need any adjustments for a quite a while. Now she just needs maintenance care from her loving husband.

My hope in sharing this anecdote is to point out the longevity of the pain brought about by this insult, or injury, to the atlas. I have had many patients who lived lives of daily headaches, migraines, vertigo, nausea, and radiating pains in the arms. Although they had tried all forms of therapy, this technique seemed to help in many cases. Their daily existence used to revolve around how bad their headaches or other ailments may or may not be—not much of a life in my book. Life is hard enough, especially when those you love and care about are dependent on you, yet it is even harder when you are unable to function on a day-to-day basis.

The spinal cord and brain's most vulnerable area is at the atlas, the junction of the skull and neck. When the supportive bones surrounding the brain stem area are moved beyond their limit, to put it in simple terms, they irritate what they are meant to protect. To see how nature adapts to this delicate area, observe a ram's atlas, which is twice the size of human's, which has a different shape, and purpose for its function—the ability to withstand mighty blows as their heads collide with those of other rams. At an advanced AO seminar, Dr. Sweat, the inventor of the atlas orthogonal technique, demonstrated the importance of the atlas to life by pointing out that, instinctively, "animals go to the base of the skull to kill prey." This is exactly where the atlas lies. When insults or injury occur at this important part of a person's neuroanatomy, it is easy to understand how a wide variety of symptoms can manifest, either instantly or over time.

TAKE AWAY: WITH KNOWLEDGE COMES ACCOUNTABILITY. WHEN THERE IS A TRAUMA TO THE SKULL, YOU NOW KNOW THAT THE ATLAS NEEDS TO BE PROFESSIONALLY EVALU-ATED TO MAKE SURE YOUR HEAD IS ON STRAIGHT.

Chapter Eleven

The Reality of a Crooked Head

For many people, living day in and day out is tough enough already. Dealing with an ongoing insult to neurological function that challenges your ability to process your world is a huge obstacle. Photophobia, or fear of light; audiophobia, fear of sound; and vertigo are some common complaints among many patients with their heads on crooked. Add debilitating migraines on top of all those symptoms, and it is easy to see how those who suffer from a misaligned atlas just want to stay in bed in a dark and quiet room. Their lives become centered on the question, "Is it going to be one of those days, and how do I function if it is?" They can't be loving and involved in the lives of those around them because they are not even able to take care of their own needs, much less the needs of a crying two-year-old or the frustrated husband who says, "Another night of those migraines, I can see it in your eyes."

This also takes a toll on people's livelihoods, as time off from work adds up. I had a patient, Laura, recently who missed five days of work the month before due to headaches. Not only was her head bothering her but she also did not have the strength to hold up her arms. As a beautician, Laura would give between eighteen and thirty-two haircuts per day. Not so when her head was throbbing and her arms were unable to support their own weight. Days like that she could only stay in bed and ride it out.

There are too many people in this world with their heads on crooked. For those I can treat and level out, it's rewarding to see them become more productive and functional. While evaluating a new patient, it is easy to observe someone with a marked head tilt. Although he or she may be able to shift his head from side to side, the resting position of his head will be tilted to one side. For some this may seem hard to believe, but I often tell them to look at a picture of themselves and they will see that their head is consistently tilted to one side. One ear will be higher, the center of the skull will be off toward one shoulder, and this will be the position they naturally fall into time and time again. "This is normal for me. I always do this," they say. I come back with, "That's because the only bone that supports your head is not squarely under your skull."

I began a case in the spring of 2016 as a referral from a local doctor of Osteopathy. Caroline was brutally assaulted by a disgruntled boyfriend in the fall of 2004. At the hospital she was told she was lucky to be alive. In a four-page testimonial, Caroline would later write,

> The trauma to my neck left it completely unable to lift or even hold my head up and [it] took several months to regain [the] strength to do so. Throughout the years, I suffered with head, neck, and body pain and the pain got progressively worse....Years of blood work, MRIs with and without contrast, CAT scans, neck and spine x-rays revealed nothing.

The blows and kicks to Caroline's head had caused the first bone in her neck (the atlas) to become misaligned. The result of that deviation under her skull made it impossible for her to function. Caroline would wake up in pain, and that would structure her entire day. The longest of her migraines lasted two solid weeks. She had vertigo, photophobia, audiophobia, and she was often nauseated. She was unable to perform daily tasks and was so overwhelmed with medical issues that finding a job was unimaginable. It became a struggle just for her to walk a short distance. Before beginning care at our clinic, Caroline was well into the process of applying for disability aid from the government, after ten-plus years of leading such a handicapped life.

We took X-rays of Caroline's upper neck and found that her atlas had displaced to the right side of her skull by more than six millimeters and had rotated backward by more than six degrees. An average misalignment at my clinic is typically one to three millimeters of lateral deviation and less than two degrees of rotation. This deviation was causing irritation to her brain stem, and this is why she was having such a barrage of symptoms.

I adjusted her atlas with the Atlas Orthogonal Percussion Instrument, Dr. Roy Sweat's invention. Caroline said the procedure seemed like "a burst of air and I didn't feel a thing." Later, she wrote:

> The biggest changes started to happen shortly after that visit. I slept all night without taking a sleeping pill and did not wake up once. The most amazing thing was getting out of bed the next morning and not [needing] a pain pill.
>
> My children have also benefitted from this because they have their mommy back. I am actively searching for employment again and feel so eager to return. That is something I thought was impossible.

One reason she felt that much better was the instantaneous change that took place around her brain stem. When the atlas misaligns (subluxates), it shifts away from its perfect placement under the skull, going higher on one side. At the same time, it will twist ether forward or backward. This poor woman had had her head so badly twisted by the kicks to her skull that the atlas was rotated backward by over six degrees. Once we adjusted her, the rotation of her atlas came down to less than one degree and the lateral displacement came down to less than two millimeters! Those whose atlases are twisted to a greater degree suffer the most severe neurological injuries.

Picture the analogy of your thumb pads pressing against each other again. If you also imagine a line connecting those right and left pads at the front and back, you will have a pretty good idea of the shape of the atlas, that ring of bone surrounding your brain stem. When it rotates, the stress created at the top travels right down the spinal cord to the end, called the *filum terminale*, or "horse tail," in Greek. That is a good name for the anatomy because the spinal cord fractions off like hairs at the bottom of the spine as it goes down each leg. The twisting that begins at the top comes to an abrupt stop at the bottom, for there is no room for twisting there. Patients with severe atlas misalignments, in addition to having upper neck pain, headaches, and all the malaise that accompanies brain stem irritation, are often plagued with central low-back pain that is ongoing, like Caroline suffered.

Attending a business-after-hours meeting through our chamber of commerce, I started a conversation with a manager of the Best Western hotel. She was looking for some good front desk help. I shared that opportunity with Caroline, and after three weeks on the job she was promoted to manager! Instead of relying on the government for support, she is now contributing back to society and getting back to her life.

It's patients like Caroline that I dreamed about helping while I was a student at Life University. Practicing chiropractic day in and day out is about helping people who had just been surviving because they could not find the help they needed and seeing them be healed. Hopefully this book will give the reader hope for themselves or a loved one that there is an answer to the nagging complaints of their bodies. To look beyond the simple answer of just popping a pill for some normalcy in life and help people truly understand what is going on in their bodies is a pathway I love to help people walk down. True relief comes from addressing the cause of a problem. Fortunately for Caroline, her path eventually led to my clinic, where we applied atlas orthogonal care, and once her head was on straight, her entire life changed. If you or someone you love is suffering from neurological insult, then I urge you to consult with a board certified atlas orthogonalist to get your or your loved ones head on straight and get your life back.

TAKE AWAY: As Daniel David Palmer, the founder of chiropractic therapy, said, "There is a vast difference between treating the effects and treating the cause."

Chapter Twelve

A History of AO

The art and science of atlas orthogonal chiropractic is the study of the spine with specific concentration on the first bone in the neck, the atlas vertebrae. This bone was named for the Greek god, Atlas, who carried the world on his shoulders. The atlas bone carries your world on its shoulders by supporting your skull. A conventional chiropractic adjustment is done with the doctor's hands, but atlas orthogonal chiropractic utilizes a precise, repeatable, X-ray-analyzed chiropractic program to adjust the atlas vertebrae with the percussive force instrument invented by Dr. Roy Sweat to remove nerve interference.

As practically all chiropractors agree, the atlas is one unique and important bone to have in alignment. This importance was first singled out by Dr. B.J. Palmer. Being the first chiropractor to demonstrate this importance, Palmer is considered one of the first great atlas chiropractors. He oversaw many seemingly miraculous cases in which the patients were healed of many conditions due to the atlas being correctly adjusted. In his study of some five thousand patients, he documented changes from arthritis to asthma, from sciatica to sinusitis.

B.J. Palmer—the son of D.D. Palmer, the father of chiropractic—graduated from his father's school, Palmer College of Chiropractic, in 1902. His wife, Mabel, graduated from the school in 1905. A well-respected physician, Palmer is remembered as a leading citizen in Davenport, Iowa, where the plaque reads, "B.J. Palmer, world renowned as spokesman-developer of his father's discovery of chiropractic. Famed educator, traveler, author, radio-television pioneer (WOC-radio and TV), among the nation's first. President, Palmer College of Chiropractic, 1905–1961."[37]

By the 1920s, the school's enrollment was over two thousand students, far exceeding the number studying at other schools. Not only did B.J. practice and teach chiropractic, but in 1922 he bought a radio station he named Wonders of Chiropractic (WOC). Among the announcers he hired was a young man named Ronald Reagan who wanted to become a Hollywood hero and wound up being the fortieth president of the United States.[38] B.J. was no stranger to politics and is credited with traveling extensively to successfully introduce legislation and fight more court battles than anyone else to improve the profession. He was president of the International Chiropractors Association from 1926 until his death in 1961. One saying credited to B.J. is "Early to bed, early to rise, work like hell, and advertise, makes a man healthy, wealthy and wise," a philosophy he practiced as well as preached.[39] He also said, "The world makes a path for the man who knows where he is going"[40] and "To take a new idea you must first destroy the old, let go of old opinions, to observe and conceive new thoughts. To learn is but to change your opinion."[41]

B.J. corrected atlases using his hands (a technique called toggling), exerting up to forty pounds of pressure on the bone. This technique became standard practice for many years. The atlas vertebrae differ from all other spinal segments in a variety of ways. First off, it is the most mobile unit in the whole spine,

---

[37] Rondberg, *Chiropractic First*, 16.

[38] Ibid., 18.

[39] Ibid., 19.

[40] Ibid.

[41] "B. J. Palmer Quotes," *AZ Quotes*, www.azquotes.com/author/21536-B_J_ Palmer?p=2.

with "forty-seven degrees of rotation left or right."[42] The axis vertebra is the largest bone of the cervical spine and is located directly beneath the atlas. The atlas is the lightest segment of the twenty-four moveable bones making up the spine. It has no connecting disc under it, as do the other twenty-three. In its uniqueness, it does not have interlocking joints, called facets, like all the other segments. Through extensive study, Palmer figured out the importance of adjusting the atlas from the side; adjusting it via the transverse process of the vertebrae was the better way to deliver the corrective force. Palmer later taught students such as Dr. Sweat to adjust the atlas on the transverse process of that bone using a side posture table. That's the part of your atlas you put your fingertip on back in Chapter Ten.

The next great upper cervical doctor to further the understanding of atlas correcting, realizing that less force is needed to make an adjustment, was Dr. John Grostic. Another student of Palmer's, Grostic was credited with, while still using his hands for adjusting, utilizing a lot less force to make the correction. In 1947 Dr. Roy Sweat began studying at the Palmer College with B.J. Palmer. Sweat became interested in the field of chiropractic after seeing his sister's improvement from the migraines she had suffered from for many years when a chiropractor adjusted her atlas. Sweat later studied under Grostic, and by 1957 Sweat was teaching with Grostic. In their in-depth clinical research, Grostic and Sweat found that significantly less force could be used to correct the atlas position. The pair also noticed the differences in students' abilities to toggle the atlases of their patients. This observation prompted Sweat to build a machine that would allow chiropractors of all sizes and strengths to adjust the atlas equally.

---

[42] Augustus A. White III and Manohar M. Panjabi, *Clinical Biomechanics of the Spine* (Philadelphia, PA: J. B. Lipponcott, 1978), 65.

Sweat realized the need for a way to deliver that corrective adjustment that could be repeated independent of the chiropractor. He found that there were just too many variables to consistently accomplish a correct atlas adjustment. Whether the doctor coming to the table has a lumberjack body and weighs 350 pounds or is a petite female coming in at just under 100 pounds, all doctors need to have the same ability to apply pressure to the atlas. To address this need, Sweat developed a highly sophisticated instrument—the Atlas Orthogonal Percussion Instrument—that is capable of accurately repositioning the atlas vertebra without pain or stress.

The Atlas Orthogonal Percussion Instrument, which looks like a sci-fi movie prop, creates a percussion wave or vibration to accomplish the task of adjusting the atlas in a far more precise and gentle manner than toggling. "All doctors are equal who use the atlas orthogonal technique," Sweat said. "New students can adjust as well as I can. That's the way it should be." The Georgia Institute of Technology's engineering department helped Dr. Sweat develop, define, and refine the X-ray vector program of adjusting. Seven versions of the AO instrument have been updated for precision and excellence over the years. And since the development of the AO instrument, there have been numerous books and articles on the subject.

Sweat began teaching his procedure in the 1970s and is still teaching today at Life University as well as other colleges. I not only had the privilege of being taught by Sweat but also to now call him my friend. To actually sit and be taught by a man who was taught by the son of our profession's founder from the nineteenth century was a humbling event. At that time in my professional development, I was delivering adjustments of up to 40 to 60 pounds of thrust into that two- to three-ounce bone called the atlas—and getting some pretty good results at that. Yet, something Dr. Matt Sweat, the son of Dr. Roy Sweat, said stuck with me: "Lighter is righter." Although grammatically he was off the mark, something in that simple sentence has a chord of truth in it.

Dr. Sweat, now ninety years old, says of his percussion instrument, "I wouldn't still be working if I was still adjusting by hand." And work he still does—passionately, six days a week to make sure this line of health care is propagated to help people get their heads on straight. The knowledge gleaned from The R.W. Sweat Foundation's research studies has helped millions of patients and their families, students, and doctors over the years. At the end of every seminar and most phone calls, with a fatherly tone, the Atlanta-based physician says to fellow atlas orthogonalists, "We need you out there," to which I reply, "We need you down there in Atlanta."[43] Sweat says there is always room for improvement, and he is glad to see so many people studying the atlas. He noted that at least half of today's chiropractors incorporate therapy and nutrition into their treatments. "There are 6.5 billion people on earth and they all need a chiropractic exam. Most of them need their atlases adjusted," Sweat said.

In today's AO clinic, the first step in all cases is the taking of a history followed by an examination. Depending on the examination findings, X-rays are then taken to define the degree to which the atlas is unbalanced. Once this is known, the doctor develops a course of treatment and delivers the first adjustment. Here is where the fine detail work comes into play. Laying the patient on his or her side on an AO adjusting table, the AO doctor then places the patient's head upon a special section of the table called the headpiece. The doctor's job is to take all the stress of the skull off the atlas while at the same time creating a subtle pull on the bones of the neck via muscles and ligaments. A slender metal tube, called the stylus, is placed over the atlas. When the instrument is triggered, a vibration travels down the

---

[43] See Appendix B for an interview with Dr. Sweat.

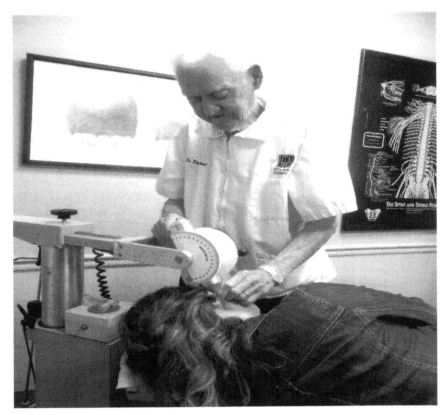

Atlas Orthogonal Adjustment
6 pounds

Dr. Roy Sweat adjusting with the Atlas Orthogonal Percussion Instrument.

stylus, going right into the atlas and causing it to shift back into alignment. This correction is due to the detailed placement of stresses positioned upon the upper neck while a precise corrective force realigns the atlas. Finally, another set of X-rays will be taken to analyze the change.

Atlas orthogonal chiropractic is now taught at five chiropractic colleges and is practiced in six countries and in more than six hundred chiropractic clinics worldwide. Medical doctors, neurologists, podiatrists, endocrinologists, dentists, and other chiropractors refer their patients to atlas orthogonal chiropractor because they know atlas orthogonal chiropractic adjustment is safe, painless, and full of incredible results and that your upper cervical spine is vital to your health and well-being. In the following chapters, we'll explore some of the benefits of AO in greater depth.

TAKE AWAY: AS OUR UNDERSTANDING OF THIS HIGHLY SEN-SITIVE NEUROLOGICAL AREA DEVELOPS, PATIENTS SHOULD SEEK OUT PRACTITIONERS WHO APPLY THIS UNDERSTAND-ING AND GET RESULTS.

Chapter Thirteen

Traumas to the Neck

Old stories from the West tell how a condemned man would be set upon his horse with a noose around his neck. The end of the rope would be tied to an overhanging tree branch and the horse spooked—to its owner's demise. Though this may sound harsh, it was actually a more merciful method for this form of execution. A common misconception about hanging is that it causes death by strangulation. But, if death were to be caused by strangling, it would be a pretty gruesome event. The condemned could be kicking on the end of the rope up to seven minutes before he or she died from asphyxiation. The cause of death from a proper hanging is the severing of the spinal cord at the brain stem. When the condemned dropped down and the hangman's noose jolted taut, the head was thrown forward while the single strand of rope in the front lurched backward. That forward and backward motion at the exact junction of the skull resting upon the atlas forced the bones of the upper neck to rip from their resting places, tearing into the brain stem. Often, the prisoner would be dead before he stopped bouncing. In essence, hanging serves the purpose of the medieval guillotine—but without the mess.

The hanging process is similar, to varying degrees, to what happens in whiplash accidents that affect more than one million drivers each year. In automobiles, the purpose of the head-rest is to stabilize the skull and upper neck to prevent injury in the event of an accident. The following illustration shows what can and does happen when a car is struck in the rear, unless the driver's head is resting on the headrest at the moment of impact. The human skull weights between nine and eighteen pounds; therefore, let's imagine a twelve-pound bowling ball as an example. Picture the bowling ball sitting there in an old Pinto, perfectly still, a good six to ten inches away from the headrest, dreaming of that perfect three-hundred-point game. *Wham*! A 4,000-pound car hits from behind, striking the bowling ball's bumper at a speed of 30 miles an hour. The force (*force* equals *mass* times *acceleration*, or $F = M \times A$) of that stationary car our happy bowling ball was daydreaming in is now traveling less than 30 miles an hour toward the back of that ball. The mass of the 4,000-pound car multiplied by the speed of 30 miles an hour will result in a massive force that will impact the bowling ball (or head).

It is widely believed that the true damage in whiplash cases happens in the nanosecond of impact. That is when the force (F) is applied to the soft tissue that supports and gives function to our bowling ball, causing the most damage. The medical term for this type of lasting injury to the soft tissue is called ligament laxity; if it is secondary to injuries sustained in a whiplash injury, it could prove to be life altering. In the neck, if the vertebrae go beyond three to five millimeters in normal range of motion on X-rays, it is classified as a Category IV permanent impairment of 25 to 28 percent whole person (i.e., a loss of 25 to 28 percent of medical functionality), according to American Medical Association (AMA) guidelines.[44] This means that the ligaments of the neck are so torn or damaged that they cannot do their job of supporting and maneuvering the skull. You need to be able to hold your skull in a desired position and move it into the next desired position.

---

[44] Steven Eggleston, "Accurate Prognosis in Personal-Injury Cases Using George's Line," *Dynamic Chiropractic* 28, no. 7 (March 26, 2010).

Two of my patients come to mind in this context. Both were involved in pretty forceful accidents. One was a rear-end accident case, the other a side impact. Both had had other chiropractic care before coming to my clinic and did improve some with the atlas orthogonal work but not entirely. Prior to the rear-end impact, one patient was an active runner; suffice it to say she is not up and running. She has gone the medical route, trying to surgically correct her problem, but unfortunately her neck was so severely damaged that the instability could not be corrected by any health care professional. The other one has repeatedly asked me to never move, for she wants to be under my care for the rest of her life, being seen once every two to three weeks. Her life has gotten back to close to where it once was, yet due to the damage she will never have the stability of a normal neck.

The development of modern automobiles has come a long way—possibly too far. In improving the design of newer cars, the automotive industry's focus was on making the automobile more durable. Funny, this trails back to money. In the 1970s, insurance companies started complaining about damages to the automobile during low-impact crashes. They complained loudly enough to get the government to start passing laws demanding that car manufactures build cars that don't crumple easily upon impact. Let's get back to physics for a moment: $F = M \times A$. Although the cars would not be damaged, the force (F) is still going somewhere. If the rear bumper does not cave in in response to the force, that impact is going to be dispersed within the car, including its occupants. Often the maxim "no crash, no cash" is falsely applied. The logic behind it is, if the car shows no damage, how can the driver make a claim that he was hurt (although the injuries can be severe)? What's your take?

Automobile accident research has taken the formula $F = M \times A$ to the next level, incorporating Delta V (velocity) over Delta

T (time).[45] The ambitious reader may want to consult the references to get a better grasp of this formula, but for the purposes of this book, suffice it to say that the speed, or decrease of speed, over a certain period of time is where the "rubber meets the road." My nephew, who is pretty sharp, explained the significance of Delta V over Delta T in this analogy: Two people stand side by side on top of a one-story building. They both jump off at the same time. The first jumper—we'll call him the smarter of the two—lands with his knees bent. This softens the blow to his body and, at a scientific level, allows the force upon impact to travel through his body over a longer period of time. The other guy lands with his knees locked. From a scientific perspective, the force of impact would therefore go through his body in a shorter period of time. Besides causing damage to his knees, hips, and low back, there is a good chance that this foolhardy guy even misaligned his atlas as that additional stress went racing through his body.

In cars with stiffer bumpers, therefore, the metal of the car does not collapse in response to the force of impact, and the stress of the impact goes through the car at a much faster rate. In rear-end accidents where the bumper and trunk don't crumple, that force goes somewhere real fast—often into the driver's body. In one study, researchers found that a change in velocity (Delta V) in accidents of less than 9.3 miles per hour caused an injury rate of 36 percent. Yet, in accidents at speeds higher than 9.3 miles per hour, the injury rate is only 20 percent. Because the faster speeds would typically cause greater crumpling or damage to the car, research reveals that there is actually less injury

45 J. Y. Foret-Bruno, F. Dauvilliers, C. Tarriere, and P. Mack, "Influence of the Seat and Head Rest Stiffness on the Risk of Cervical Injuries," study presented at the 13th International Technical Conference on Experimental Safety Vehicles, November 4–7, 1991, Paris, France (Washington, DC: The National Academies of Sciences, Engineering, and Medicine Transportation Research Board, 1993), 68, https://trid.trb.org/view.aspx?id=409157.

to vehicle occupants for rear-end accidents at higher speeds.[46] A 16 percent difference is pretty significant in my book.

I am just north of six foot two. When I get in a car, I like to make sure the headrest height is appropriate for my height so that it serves its purpose. If I am ever rear-ended, regardless of the speed at impact, I want the back of my skull to make contact with the headrest. If my skull is just above that support, my twelve-pound bowling ball is going to lurch backward at X miles per hour and the atlas area will be left to deal with all that shearing force. To go back to "Neuroanatomy 101," there is no bony contact on our bowling ball, only soft tissue, and if that headrest is not supporting the head, the soft tissue has to tolerate all that stress. That soft tissue is comprised of over a dozen muscles with ligaments that attach the skull to the neck, and of course all the nerves that give function to your body.

Of course, one needn't experience anything as severe as the trauma of an accident to knock the atlas out of alignment. In fact, I recently treated a patient with a most unusual cause of insult. I began treating this female patient for bad headaches in October 2011. Her therapy has had good results; I have adjusted her atlas only six times within a six-year period. The odd thing was, her misalignment had changed from the left side to the right side, as evident in the X-rays we took. Although I knew from the X-rays that she had changed from a left-side to a right-side atlas misalignment, which typically doesn't happen, I didn't know how it happened. Because a major impact like that of a car accident or a blow to the skull can make that change, I asked her if she had hit her head on something. She wasn't holding her adjustment as she should, and the resulting vertigo had gotten so bad that she was unable to even lie down on her back for a leg-length check. As it turns out, the culprit of her "trauma" was her two-and-a-half-year-old son. At the age of six months, this little guy had

---

[46] Ibid.

started clinging to his momma's right earlobe, pulling it down toward his head for ten to fifteen minutes at a time. Sure, this made her neck a little stiff, but being the good mother that she is, she gave in to her little boy's desire. She had done this whenever she laid him down for a nap or to bed for the night—for the past two years! The continual, daily stress of that positioning over two years could and had changed her misalignment.

I once had a massage therapist who worked in my clinic. I warned her about the importance of being mindful of the upper cervical area in her work. However, in performing a massage, she put so much pressure just under the skull that she caused a patient's atlas misalignment to shift from the left side to the right side of her neck. This shift was made possible because when one is lying face down on a massage table, totally relaxed, and someone applies pressure just under the skull, the posterior arch of the atlas is very vulnerable. There are no locking joints, there's no disc, it's the lightest bone in the spine, and the neck muscles are not firing to protect it because the person is lying down. When this particular massage therapist did this a second time, I fired her.

One last point to bring home: I often hear my female patients complain of experiencing neck pain or headaches when they get their hair washed at the beauty parlor. Usually it stems from the point when they lay their heads back in the basin to wash and rinse. The edge of the basin is often too narrow to give their bowling ball the support it needs, and the thin, back portion of the atlas bears all that weigh and stress. Even this temporary stress to that light bone can cause it to shift slightly, resulting in some of the problems discussed throughout this book.

TAKE AWAY: IF YOU WANT TO AVOID NECK TRAUMA, MAKE SURE YOU ELEVATE THE HEADREST IN YOUR CAR, HAVE A NEUROLOGICAL CONSULTATION WITH YOUR MASSEUSE, AND, IF YOUR BEAUTICIAN'S BASIN FEELS LIKE A GUILLO-TINE, USE A TOWEL TO CUSHION THE CONTACT.

Chapter Fourteen

Traumatic Brain Injury (TBI)

As God would have it, I moved to a small city in eastern North Carolina that is home to a traumatic brain injury center called ReNu Life. I seized the opportunity to see if I could be of help to some of the residents. According to the Centers for Disease Control and Prevention (CDC), "In 2013, about 2.8 million TBI-related emergency department (ED) visits, hospitalizations, and deaths occurred in the United States."[47] In 1980 I was one of those statistics. Now I serve on the board of the Brain Injury Association of North Carolina (BIANC). There are 3.1 million people living with long-term disability as a result of TBI. I often wonder how many of them are still suffering from a misaligned atlas. Not only does the atlas misalign, it often becomes fixated in that misaligned position. That is the area in which I can give my patients hope: hope that I can give them relief from an insult to the brain stem due to a misaligned atlas. This hope makes adjusting and realigning the atlas the focus of my practice. The reality of what I have seen clinically in my dozen-plus years of doing this work causes me to pause and reflect back. To sum it up, in view of the time of the trauma and when and if corrective care at the brain stem begins, I see the atlas subluxation as an undiagnosed and untreated causative factor in many ongoing

---

[47] "TBI: Get the Facts," *Centers for Disease Control and Prevention*, April 27, 2017, www.cdc.gov/traumaticbraininjury/get_the_facts.html.

ailments, such as migraines, vertigo, and insomnia, just to list a few.

The vast majority of TBI cases—I would say 98 percent or more—are due to physical trauma. The other 2 percent are due to chemical or drug reactions. The event that causes a physical blow to the skull can vary, from a fall from a high chair, a skateboard, or a roof top. It could be caused by the force of impact against a dashboard in a high-speed car crash or from simply hitting the ground as a person's body surrenders to gravity from some reason.

The CDC reports that falls are the number one cause of TBIs.[48] The cause of these falls could be as simple as a person, oftentimes elderly, tripping over something in the dark or, as in my case, as traumatic as the skull hitting the ground after being catapulted over the handlebars of a motorcycle, resulting in a great force being applied to the skull. In layman's terms, your brain gets rattled. And in such cases, that two- to three-ounce bone called the atlas is no longer in its correct place.

The inventor of the technique of atlas orthogonal, Dr. Roy Sweat, states, "When a force enters through the lower body it will travel up the spinal segments until it hits the atlas; due to its small size, it is unable to transmit the force, causing that bone to displace." As we know, the atlas is a two- to three-ounce bone and the skull is like a bowling ball, weighing nine to seventeen pounds. Inversely, blows to the head will cause this force to travel down the spine, causing the same phenomena as a hit to the lower body. The atlas (represented anatomically as C-1) sits on top of the axis (C-2), the largest bone in the cervical spine, often causing the insult to remain just under the skull—a real "pain in the neck."

I will state the obvious, yet I wonder why it is not addressed by the medical profession because it is so sensible: *The force it takes to actually crack a human skull is many*

---

[48] Ibid.

times greater than the force that would cause the most mobile joint in the spine to move beyond its normal limits. **So, too, in concussions. When the force of trauma to the skull is great enough to bring about a concussion, then one needs to look just under the skull, at the atlas, for an injury there as well. A good saying that should be in all ER facilities is, "With a blow to the skull, look just below."** I once treated a patient whose skull had been crushed in. He suffered with debilitating migraines for over a decade before he came to be under my care. A logical deduction that I want to point out here is that, even before the plates of the skull crush in upon the brain cavity, that force is going to result in a shifting of the atlas vertebrae from its neutral position underneath the skull.

Of course, I am using an extreme example, but the point I am trying to make here is that even with a relatively minor jolt to the head, as in the time that I bumped my own noggin in my clinic, the Occipital Atlanto Axial articulation (that's medical jargon for where your skull sits on your neck) can be disrupted. This causes dysfunction of that ever-so-important joint, evidenced by a list of symptoms that include migraine headaches, nausea, and vertigo, among many others. However, one common warning sign is simply a stiff neck. Having the ability to look to one side but not equally to the other is an indication that something is not quite right. Although there are seven bones in the neck and atlas rotation accounts for 58 percent of neck rotation, if the atlas is not aligned perfectly, then that is your limitation. As AO chiropractors, we always check patients' leg lengths and palpate their necks before we make an adjustment. The leg lengths show us whether or not the spine has twisted or muscles have contracted to compensate for the misalignment of the atlas. Almost invariably, the upper neck will have very sore and painful nodules. Those sore spots will be found just below your mastoid process at the base of the skull.

I had one patient, Desirae, from Jamaica. Desirae had bilateral tender spots just below her skull. I scanned them by palpitation (feeling with the fingers) just before the correction, placed her down on her side, and adjusted her atlas. Sitting her back up, I rescanned her neck and, with a smile nearly as wide as her face, she said, "Dhat's magic!" Desirae could not believe the pain in her neck was gone that quickly. When I palpated her neck, I too felt the irritation was gone. Another patient, upon her first adjustment, said, "Don't tell my husband, but I love you!" Although I graduated more than thirty years ago, one of my favorite experiences is still adjusting a new patient's atlas for the first time. Their immediate response to the correction affirms in my heart that, yes, I am making a positive difference in the lives of others.

Allow me to explain leg lengths now. I vividly recall an Advance AO seminar at which we had an ophthalmologist explain to us that the eye will actually rotate in its socket three to five degrees to compensate for crooked heads. For greater misalignments, the whole body has to adapt to balance out that crooked head. That adaptation is done by one leg pulling up shorter than the other.

The case of Ricky gives us an example of why leg lengths matter. Ricky is one of the residents at ReNu Life. He is a gentle giant who came to my clinic for the first time at age thirty-one. All of his shoes had had the left sole built up three-fourths of an inch higher than the right due to the difference in his leg length.

On November 17, 1994, at the age of fourteen, Ricky was riding his bike from his home to a nearby convenience store. It was a trip he had made many times. A car hit him from behind, flipping Ricky straight up. When Ricky came down, he landed on the roof of the car, striking his skull and crushing it. Surgeons had to pull out pieces of Ricky's skull and drain the blood and excessive fluid from his head. They then inserted a monitor to keep watch on the amount of pressure his brain received from inflammation and bleeding. He underwent a tracheotomy and was breathing through a tube. The boy spent the next two months in a coma and remained hospitalized until March 1995. He had profound memory impairment. Arriving home, Ricky's parents noticed the difference in the lengths of his legs. His doctors explained it away as a one-sided growth spurt. Having no better explanation—and probably at their wits' ends by this time—Ricky's parents arranged for his special shoes.

He became my patient on May 11, 2011. An examination of Ricky revealed that he did in fact have an atlas misalignment. The only bone that was supporting Ricky's head was jammed up to the left side of his skull, preventing his head from coming back into balance. Ricky did not have a one-sided growth spurt; his head was crooked and his body had adapted to that deviation. The difference in his leg length was an indication of his body's innate intelligence, which was trying to level out his head.

Innate intelligence controls and regulates all aspects of living. It is what directs the blood flow away from those stiff blue digits that are going through a severe case of frostbite. If your body was still pumping blood to those fingers and toes, keeping them warm and comfy, then your core temperature would drop and your "innards" would get blue and stiff. Many professionals believe innate intelligence to be God's overriding control of His greatest creation.

After his first adjustment, Ricky's head became centered over his body for the first time in seventeen years. Now I was in a pickle. Was I to allow my patient to walk out of my clinic with an unnecessary three-quarter-inch shoe lift, or have him walk out in his socks? I chose the latter and have that pair of his shoes as a keepsake.

Ricky now has a much better chance at doing what we take for granted, his gait improved right away. His sense of balance is grounded. A lot of his postural distortions that were brought

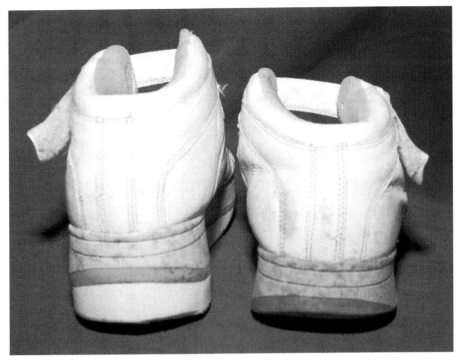

Ricky's custom-built shoes.

Photo Credit: Calvin N. Sanders, C&B Photography LLC

on by his body's struggle to level off his head were no longer needed. To simply stand upright now took a lot less effort. The joy and fulfilled hope that comes to life so quickly upon clearing out irritation at such a critical neurological location is why I am so passionate about this line of work. That adjustment that I had given Ricky changed him in such a profound and life-altering way that I only wish it could have happened sooner.

In studying the way our bodies react to leveling out our heads, I came across some interesting information. Roger Sperry, the 1981 Nobel Prize winner for brain research, is often quoted as saying, "Better than 90 percent of the energy output of the brain is used in relating to the physical body in its gravitational field. The more mechanically distorted a person is, the less energy available for thinking, metabolism, and healing." View that statement in line with the mechanical/neurological distortion that comes about due to atlas displacement. I like to share a computer analogy with my patients. Say you are using a computer with only one program running, compared to a similar model that has fifteen programs running. Which one is going to run better? So, too, is it with our bodies. If your brain is firing off extra muscles just to allow you to stand erect, then, in my book, that is wasted brain power.

TAKE AWAY: ANY IDEA WHAT THE NUMBER-ONE ACTIVITY IS THAT CAUSES TBIS? IT'S NOT FOOTBALL, SOCCER, OR EVEN BOXING. WOULD YOU BELIEVE IT'S BICYCLE RIDING! IF YOU OR YOUR LOVED ONES HAVE BICYCLES, YOU BETTER HAVE HELMETS TOO.

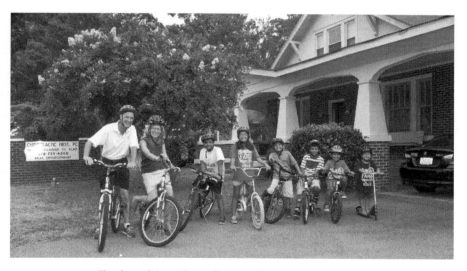

Dr. Gallagher, his wife and a number of their godchildren.

Photo Credit: Calvin N. Sanders, C&B Photography LLC

Chapter Fifteen

Sleep and AO

Chiropractors may not run ads during the Super Bowl, but we continually tell our patients to seek the root of the problem before jumping to the quick, and often temporary, fix of medication. This approach is not in the public consciousness, and they need to be made aware of it. A topic I address in my talks with new patients and their families centers on the question, are we understanding the signals of our bodies? The TV commercials say, "These signals are an indication our product is needed." Since 1895, with the invention of chiropractic, the chiropractic profession has been saying, "Correct the body's complaint. Don't just medicate it." But sometimes people don't realize that misalignment can cause neurological problems. Take, for instance, a person's ability to sleep. Despite the abundance of sleep aids on the market, oftentimes an off-centered atlas is to blame.

Many people don't know that when you rush to get out of your car and knock your head against the doorjamb and your neck gets stiff right away, a good night's sleep might not do the trick. Even so, if the person cannot get a good night's sleep, then that is often a sign that something is not quite right. Furthermore, when sleep becomes elusive, a host of other symptoms, like headaches, fatigue, irritability, and vertigo, begin a barrage of insults to your central nervous system.

Olivia, a patient in one of my clinics, was ready to undergo a sleep study to learn why she was having so much difficulty falling asleep. After her first adjustment—no study needed—she found the answer: her head was on crooked! She was on a "pillow of needles" when trying to find that comfortable spot where she could doze off. The irritation just under her skull would not allow her to sleep comfortably; no matter how many times she turned, how often she fluffed up her pillow, or how many sheep she counted, she could not find peaceful slumber. The problem was not how her head was placed upon her pillow but how her head was placed upon her body—that being not orthogonal! (*Orthogonal* is Greek for being at a ninety-degree angle from one part to another.)

I often tell my new patients, just after their first atlas adjustment, "Some of the responses you may sense are better breathing, energy levels, digestion, and sleep. The most notable one is sleep. People know when they have a good night's sleep and inversely they know when they don't have a good night's sleep. A good REM (Rapid Eye Movement) sleep is the time period within a twenty-four-hour day when we do a lot of internal R&R to help our bodies stay healthy and function optimally in this busy world we live in.

I once had a case involving a ten-year-old girl. Kathleen had been my patient for over a year. Recently, she was playing soccer at her church and suddenly got knocked in the head. Subsequently, Kathleen developed headaches and failed to find that restful spot that allows for a great night's sleep. Her mother, JoAnne, had been my patient even longer, and the "mom knows best" instinct kicked in, so she brought her daughter to my clinic within days of the injury. Sure enough, Kathleen's atlas was misaligned to the left side and twisted backward under her skull.

After I adjust a patient's atlas, he or she is required to take a mandatory ten-minute rest on one of our tables. This young girl stretched out for her rest period. But a gentle nudge and a comment, "Your time's up," failed to wake her. I had to carry her out to the family's SUV to begin the two-hour ride home. Kathleen slept the whole way because her head was put back on straight and her body knew what it needed: rest!

TAKE AWAY: PSALMS 4:8 SAYS, "I WILL LIE DOWN AND SLEEP IN PEACE FOR YOU ALONE, OH LORD, MAKE ME DWELL IN SAFETY" (NIV). THAT VERSE, AND HAVING YOUR HEAD ON STRAIGHT, AFFORDS ONE A GOOD NIGHT'S SLEEP.

Chapter Sixteen

Why Atlas Orthogonal?

Eight Cases of Far-Reaching Neurological Consequences

In this chapter, I will present eight different cases that show what can happen when there is an ongoing stress at the brain stem level.[49] What is particularly noteworthy are the changes these patients experienced as they responded to this unique type of care. It's important to note that chiropractors don't cure anything; the two tenets of chiropractic are:

1. The body is self-healing.
2. The body is controlled by the nervous system.

To put it in a nutshell, if something is interfering with your nervous system, then your body cannot achieve the optimal outcome in its quest to be healthy. Removing that neurological insult is the act we as chiropractors do that allows the following miracles to happen.

Nancy: Multiple Sclerosis

Nancy came to our clinic in the fall of 2008. She came in on a cane and was anticipating getting a wheelchair in the near

---

[49] All testimonials have been reprinted here either with the permission of the patient or with names that have been changed.

future. The medication she was taking to halt the advance of MS was not doing much at all. After removing the interference at her brain stem, her body started to function the way God had intended. Not only did we help her put aside her walking cane, she soon showed me the photos of her hiking up a steep volcanic terrain in Hawaii with her family. Here is Nancy's testimonial, written December 17, 2008:

> Dear Dr. Gallagher,
>
> This chapter started on September 17, 2008, when I went to a church sponsored Health Fair. I received a free assessment to [your clinic] so...I went and my life was changed by your skill.
>
> I have spent years of accepting a slow downward spiral that is the usual for multiple sclerosis. This diagnosis has been hanging over my head for twenty years (since 1989). I had developed a lot of the handicaps and warning signs of MS. Once multiple MRI brain scans had confirmed the benchmark signs, I had resigned myself to that lifestyle. BUT...Once I learned that my head was eighteen degrees off, and Dr. Gallagher fixed that, I have a much brighter future! I walk without a cane and am looking forward to a trip to Hawaii. I hope to do some hiking with my son and grandchildren on the mountainous volcanic terrain. I will take pictures and bring some on my return.
>
> Well, there is the short history of a life with MS and I am hoping I can convince the [local] MS self-help group to have Dr. Gallagher present a short program to the friends I have there. I know that many of them could benefit from new techniques to help deal with MS.
>
> Again, I thank you for one of the greatest miracles of my life! Have a blessed holiday and I will see you in January.
>
> Yours,
>
> Nancy

Mary: TMJ

The next case describes the experience of a patient we'll call Mary. She had jaw pain that is often referred to as Temporo-mandibular Joint (TMJ) pain. As you will see, her pain was so great that life became unbearable. The irony of her story was that she was a dental hygienist, working in a profession that deals frequently with that very problem. Being a hygienist and still not being able to get relief had heightened her angst. Before coming to my clinic, she had been prescribed enough heavy-duty narcotics to put a permanent end to her pain. Her family was so concerned that she might take her own life that they tried to keep her prescription medications hidden.

When a patient leaves my clinic, I often have a good hunch whether they will respond favorably, depending on their post X-rays. These show me how much the atlas has moved back to the ideal spot under the skull. Mary's case took even me by surprise. She presented the following testimonial at her very next visit, on July 19, 2010. Although I take a pretty thorough history with new patients, sometimes I can only guess at how devastating their neurological insults are to their lives. The fact that she was possibly days away from "checking out" of the game of life serves as a reminder to me that I need to take my line of work very seriously.

> Dr. Gallagher.
>
> I wish to express my gratitude and let you know how grateful I am that you were able to help me!
>
> When I came to your office, I was at sixteen months of not eating foods that required any chewing and severe jaw pain. I had been to countless dentists, doctors, and clinics which tried to help me, but I was still not better. After all this time, I was taking many medications, narcotics, muscle relaxers, etc. Plus, receiving dental work and therapy

with no relief. One week prior to coming to your office, I was in a very dark place and was desperate with God to please show me something that would help, and felt completely hopeless.

My friend Carrie recommended I see a chiropractor that specialized with the activator and the atlas, I very reluctantly agreed to go.

After just one treatment, I felt totally different! I left your office and slept wonderfully (I had not slept good in sixteen months or more!!!), I awoke to find my jaw pain completely gone and I can now eat regular food.

Praise God and thank you so much Dr. Gallagher!!

Mary

Carl: Ear Infections

This next case serves as a reminder of just how far the standard medical profession will go to help relieve a problem that is not responding well to conventional treatment. The medical name for an ear infection is *otitis media*. Thankfully, with current research the medical community is learning that less is often better. A number of *otitis media* cases have a pretty favorable outcome if left alone, without medical intervention. Although, with children, it can be very important to correct this problem. Depending on the severity of the blockage, sound may not enter the child's perception at the developmental stage of the child's hearing. If the child is not hearing correctly, he or she will have a hard time pronouncing these sounds and forming words. Yet, one patient I treated was a teenager who had this condition since birth.

To explain what I mean by "how far the medical profession will go," consider the interventions that Carl endured before seeking chiropractic therapy. In addition to having multiple tubes placed and frequent antibiotics, Carl also underwent an uncommon surgical procedure. The word *mastoïdectomie* is not easily said and the procedure is not often performed. The medical reasoning was that this patient's ear infections might be originating from the mastoid air cell. Therefore, surgeons cut away part of Carl's skull behind both of his ears in their attempt to get rid of his lifelong ear infections—a drastic intervention that didn't seem to help. Yet, according to Carl's mother, the noninvasive natural therapy of atlas realignment worked wonders. Here is Carl's story in his mother's words:

July 29, 2009

I have a son who has been plagued with ear infections all of his life. One hundred and twenty rounds of antibiotics, four sets of ear tubes, and two mastoidectomies have all contributed to the partial hearing loss in both of his ears. So I admit that I first visited Dr. Gallagher in an act of desperation, as I had read that chiropractic treatments often help kids with ear infections, as well as kids who have autism. Yes, my son has high-functioning autism, which, strangely, is frequently accompanied by high incidences of ear infections.

Over two years ago, after fielding my emotional phone call (after yet another ear infection diagnosis!), Dr. Gallagher agreed to open his office on a Saturday morning, when he x-rayed, examined, AND adjusted my son's atlas. My son, who typically cannot describe his own physical state, moaned in relief and said, "Wow, I feel better!" I actually cried on the spot. Dr. Gallagher was very patient in working with my son, explaining to him how to not "pop" his neck, and teaching what he should and should not do to keep his neck and back in alignment. We saw Dr. G. several times afterwards, but then life went on. It took me about three months to realize that Carl did not have an ear infection, which was so unusual. Then another three months passed, but without ear infections! I could hardly believe that adjusting his atlas would so much affect my son, but it did.

Now, at age seventeen, my son has had only four infections in the past two years, which is unbelievable considering nothing could stop them before our treatments with Dr. Gallagher. He now will ask me to make an appointment when he feels that his neck is out of alignment!

I recommend this safe and effective treatment for any mother who is looking for another way of reducing her child's ear infections!

As one mother to another,

Diane

Melissa: Optic Neuritis and Multiple Sclerosis

Even within my chosen profession of chiropractic, the specialized AO technique is held in high regard. The following testimony is from a patient who is the wife of a chiropractor but who drives more than two hours to visit my clinic for AO care!

April, 15, 2016

I began seeking help from Dr. Gallagher after an episode with optic neuritis which blurred my vision. I have Multiple Sclerosis and it was the second flare up of optic neuritis I had experienced in less than one year. With the second episode of optic neuritis came a tingling in my feet that lasted eleven months. I also experienced headaches daily for years and would often wake up in the morning with a headache. I was desperate to find a natural approach to help with my symptoms.

My husband is a chiropractor so I was well aware of what wonderful things chiropractic care can do for a person. My husband suggested I see an Atlas Orthogonal practitioner. I had never been to an orthogonal chiropractor and was anxious to see if being adjusted by this technique could help my situation. My husband is very well aware of the profound effects that Atlas Orthogonal work can have in addition to full spinal care. He searched through his colleagues and Dr. Gallagher's name was presented multiple times. So I set up an appointment quickly and from the moment I met Dr. Gallagher I felt at ease. He is a very warm and compassionate person. He was excited to help me and I am so grateful for that. His office is relaxing and comfortable. This was a very stressful time in my life and I felt surrounded by people who were loving and willing to go above and beyond to help me.

After the second adjustment by Dr. Gallagher, I began to notice that my headaches had almost disappeared. I honestly can't believe that I lived so long with such constant pain. Soon after I noticed the change in my headaches, I began to see an improvement in my vision. My eyesight was something I prayed about daily and the loss of my 20/20 vision had caused me much emotional distress. I truly believe that the lack of optimal nerve flow to my eyes was a major component in my headaches and optical neuritis. By the third month under Dr. Gallagher's care, seventy-five percent of the tingling in my feet had disappeared. Although the tingling was not disabling, it was a very uncomfortable feeling and always noticeable.

I will be the first to admit I was not the easiest patient. I could not hold the adjustment at first so I had to make the drive to his office from my home more than two hours away a couple times a week for the first two months. Dr. Gallagher never gave up hope that he could help me. I cannot tell you how thankful I am to Dr. Gallagher and all his help. He is a wonderful doctor and provides an unbeliev-able service. Thank you for improving my health.

Melissa

Shearae: Equilibrium and Function

It's amazing how difficult it can be for people striving to func-tion with a neurological deficit. Things we take for granted, like equilibrium and going up and down a flight of stairs, can become practically impossible with some of these insults. The following case provides a rich example of how one patient was thrilled to now be able to do things we often take for granted.

For instance, for Shearae to navigate stairs, she could only do one step at a time, stopping each time with both feet on the same step. The true kicker in her case was that she had to lean back to compensate for her equilibrium being so off. If she were to walk down the stairs in a more upright or normal position, she would have been at risk of toppling forward. As we leveled out her atlas, her head came back to its normal position. She later commented that she only realized the difference when she was halfway down her staircase at home. She was walking nor-mally, with her head level and no fear of falling. Here is her testimonial:

> When I first came to Dr. Gallagher, I was having trouble turning my neck and rising to a standing position due to my hip mobility being slim to none in these circumstances. I also had trouble navigating stairs, having to hold on for dear life and do one step at a time due to balance issues. I had been on muscle relaxers for two years and had run out of my prescription and was in quite a bit of pain.
>
> Dr. Gallagher has me walking with more ease, standing more upright, and I have no need for the muscle relaxers. I previously was unable to sleep on my side, due to my neck

locking or getting very nauseous if I stayed on my side for more than 30-60 seconds depending on my activity that day. It made even setting my alarm a challenge, even having to take breaks.

I am happy to say, I worked in my yard last week-end. I even shoveled mulch! I also was able to lie on my side for five minutes! I only rolled over in fear of getting sick. I am very pleased and very thankful to have Dr. Gallagher and his expertise in taking the best care of me and am looking forward to being able to challenge myself further and get my life back to the appropriate level of activity!!! THANK YOU DR. GALLAGHER AND YOUR AWESOME STAFF!!

Sandy: Migraines and Nausea

This next case shows extreme results, yet it centers around a problem that a more typical patient suffers from—the dreaded headache! We BCAO doctors are frequently sought out for help dealing with migraines. Following is the testimonial offered by Sandy.

Prior to finding Dr. Patrick Gallagher, I had been suffering severe, debilitating headaches with vomiting. Medical doctors called my sickness "migraines." These headaches were daily with little let up in pain. Normally they lasted all day and night, approximately twenty-seven to twenty-nine days every month. This went on for approximately thirty years.

When the headaches were at their worst, I ended up in the hospital anywhere from three to five times a month being given oxygen, ice packs on my neck, a drug called Demerol and Morphine to stop the pain, and Phenergan to stop the vomiting. The drugs would stop the pain, but leave me so drowsy I could not function. In addition, as soon as the drugs wore off, the pain would occur again. I suffered through it and worked in pain, going into the rest-room, vomiting, and then going back to work. Many days I could not work at all. When the "migraines" started in my twenties, I went to any medical doctor I thought could help me. I had CT scans, bio-feedback, epileptic testing, brain MRI's, and other tests too numerous to list. Strange, although the doctors tested me in so many different ways, they never took x-rays of my neck.

The doctors I saw prescribed every known migraine medicine to treat me. The only thing to cut the pain and allow me to function at all was Imitrex. This drug caused my heart to race and palpitate, and caused heaviness in my chest but yet it cut the pain, so I took it anyway. The headaches were so frequent, that the nine Imitrex pills that were the normal monthly dosage didn't help much as there were more days in a month than nine. So, the doctors asked and received a waiver to up my monthly dosage to eighteen pills of Imitrex a month. That still left me with approximately twelve days where I lived in extreme pain.

About eight years ago, my cousin told me about Atlas Orthogonal Chiropractic. I searched the Internet and found Dr. Gallagher. His office was two-and-one-half hours one way from my home, but I hoped he could help me.

Dr. Gallagher took x-rays of my neck and then showed me where my atlas bone was out of alignment thereby caus-ing the extreme pain. After Dr. Gallagher set my atlas bone back in place, the headache immediately left. It was sim-ply amazing! For the first time in thirty years, I was without pain and it was without the use of pain medication!

Dr. Gallagher and the Atlas Orthogonal adjustments are my miracle from God. I now have a life free of prescribed pain medicines and one filled with absolute joy at being pain free.

I highly recommend anyone who suffers with neck or joint pain, or headaches to go see an Atlas Orthogonal Chiropractor, as you may receive your miracle too!

Blessings,

Sandy

Liam: Strep Throat and Fevers

Children's atlases and skulls are highly mobile, yet with excessive force, like falls, they too can have far-reaching neurological consequences. The following is adapted from a case study I submitted to the medical community online.[50]

One family brought their baby, Liam, to my clinic because he suffered ear infections, fevers, and difficulty in breathing and was not sleeping through the night (which is common in babies but not when the baby's sleep patterns undergo a sudden change or the problem persists night after night). The parents had tried the medication route but with limited results. Examination and X-rays revealed that the little guy's atlas had rotated backward and to the left of his skull.

Liam had been observed striking his head against a wall, which shows that the child instinctively knew that his head was off-center. His innate intelligence was to try to restore alignment and function by hitting his head against the wall. It may seem horrifying, yet his little body knew where the insult was lurking and he was trying to remove it. The child was instinctively trying to bring about homeostasis.

On Liam's first visit, we adjusted his atlas. Because labor with him had been difficult, taking twenty-four hours before

---

[50] See Appendix C for the full text of the original case study.

delivery by Cesarean section, it's possible that the baby's atlas could have been subluxated since day one. If not, a three-foot drop head first onto a concrete floor at his day care center at six months old surely was not a good thing, especially with a child since he hadn't developed his supportive neck muscles yet. When a force comes upon the skull that overwhelms the ability to maintain alignment, the skull acts like a bobble head. Yet Liam's head had bobbled too far and did not return to sit squarely over his body.

Thankfully, his rapid response to treatment is typical with children of that age. I saw Liam for a total of four visits and set his atlas only once on his first visit. Afterward, his family members noticed that he stopped hitting his head against the wall and began sleeping through the night consistently. There were no reports of fevers or ear infections, and his vocabulary was observed to have greatly improved. Children's anatomy is so dynamic at that age that their bodies are abounding with potential and energy to grow and develop.

Matthew: Cerebral Palsy

The following case covers essentially the whole life history of Matthew. He came to me as a hard-working, married man in his mid-thirties.

At two years of age, due in part to the fact that Matthew wasn't crawling well at all, he was diagnosed with Cerebral Palsy (CP). The doctors never knew exactly how the oxygen supply to his brain was disrupted, but it was. "While Cerebral Palsy (pronounced seh-ree-brel pawl-zee) is a blanket term commonly referred to as 'CP' and described by loss or impairment of motor function, Cerebral Palsy is actually caused by brain damage. The brain damage is caused by brain injury or abnormal development of the brain that occurs while a child's brain is still developing—before birth, during birth, or immediately after birth."[51]

In Matthew's case, the brain damage affected his lower limbs. To put it mildly, the message to walk was not reaching his legs. He had such spasticity that he walked on the balls of his feet, until medical doctors cut his Achilles tendons to allow his feet to go level with the ground. That was one of many operations Matthew underwent to try to correct his body.

Matthew's parents encouraged him to pursue as normal a life as was practical. He played sports. Regarding baseball, I asked, "How was your running?" "It was faster than my walking," he replied. Nevertheless, his falls were too numerous to list.

Once Matthew was riding a bicycle and went crashing over the handle bars. He was knocked unconscious and, knowing anatomy, I am willing to bet he put his atlas out of place. Matthew had lower spasticity paralysis. He could not bend his knee toward his chest. He underwent numerous operations on his legs which included cutting and lengthening other muscles and the actual breaking and rotating of his femurs. Matthew's walk, or gait, was greatly challenged. To go forward, he would lean frontward and swing his upper body to get lift to his legs, which he still does. He had done this for so long that it had begun to take a toll on his low back where it met his sacrum, or tail-bone. He was diagnosed with spinal stenosis in the spring of 2012. This is essentially the same thing as arterial stenosis, the narrowing of the blood vessels, but at the spinal canal instead and was due in great measure to his altered gait. To make matters worse, his atlas was shifted to the left side of his skull and twisted backward, making his right leg draw up a half inch.

---

[51] "Definition of Cerebral Palsy," *CerebralPalsy.org*, www.cerebralpalsy.org/about-cerebral-palsy/definition.

When Matthew began care at our clinic, he would be in such a great deal of pain that his low back would be drenched in sweat despite the fact that he began care in December, not on a hot summer day. My heart went out to this guy, who performed IT work at a local community college, which required a lot of walking all over the campus. His whole life before coming to the clinic, Matthew just had to make the best of it, and he was doing the best he could. This altered gait was because, in addition to all he had been through, his head was on crooked. The following is his take on the therapy he received and the changes he enjoyed as a result:

Back in November of 2015, my back spasms and spinal stenosis had been reaching a new level of unbearable on a daily basis. It was getting to the point where getting up and sitting down was very painful and I was nearing the point of sweating due to pain all of the time. Something had to be done so I sought out a chiropractor. The reason being is that I wasn't ready for seeking out a surgeon and medicinal treatment and intervention was starting to take its toll on me. With my Cerebral Palsy, I felt that traditional chiropractic visits would be difficult at best. My gait and wear on my body is different than most due to the spasticity and muscle tightness that I have. Up to this point, I had never heard of an AO so I was very interested in trying it out.

After the initial consultation with Dr. Gallagher, a treatment plan was put in place and for the most part I have tried to follow it. I will be honest that trying to engage my core and actively keep my lower back in alignment is still work, even almost a year later. I do feel that the work that we have been able to accomplish has been beneficial. I do not rely on the non-steroidal anti-inflammatory medication as much and when a back spasm does start to present itself, I am able to head it off before it gets flared up too much and my recovery is much sooner. Now it is more like a day instead of three or four.

I am thankful for Dr. Gallagher's work and determination to find a solution that is working for me. I feel that his work has been able to provide me with a more normal way of life that doesn't involve as much medical intervention, I feel strongly that we are extending the usefulness of my body with the work that Dr. Gallagher has done and I am very appreciative of that.

Matthew

As I said before, any good chiropractor knows it's not us, the doctors, that heal the patients but the innate intelligence located within their bodies. If a patient with a "dis-ease" process is further challenged by a neurological insult, like a subluxation of the atlas, removing the neurological insult is the point at which we can offer some profound results. In accomplishing that, the body functions better, and that is quite often miraculous.

TAKE AWAY: IF YOU OR SOMEONE YOU KNOW HAS A NEUROLOGICAL PROBLEM THAT HAS STUMPED THE NEUROLOGIST AND MEDICAL FIELD, DON'T STOP THERE, HAVE THEM OR YOURSELF CHECKED OUT BY AN ATLAS ORTHOGONAL CHIROPRACTOR.

Afterword

To God Be the Glory

I first got the idea for this book while attending one of Dr. Roy Sweat's Advanced AO seminars in Atlanta in 2006. The guest speaker was a prolific author who informed an audience of ninety BCAO chiropractors how to write their own stories. After starting the book, I floundered quite a bit. I believe my wife doubted I would ever complete the book. Yet God brought me the help I needed in a person named Susan Bowmer, who just happened to be living above my clinic in Goldsboro, North Carolina. The kicker is that she is a published author who had helped four other people complete their works.

One last divine intervention was my reunion with Dr. Frank Falowski, the first chiropractor to correctly adjust my atlas in 1983. Since he is a key player in my story, I wanted to include him. In the thirty-three years since he adjusted me, I had lost all contact with him and could not locate him. I tried looking him up through Life University and even in the yearbooks I had, but to no avail. I had given up hope and just put that aside, not giving it much more thought. Then, in 2016, I was upgrading my digital X-ray system. The salesman from South Carolina told me, "I know of a doctor in Florida who might be interested in your old CR digital X-ray unit." Once again, God did what I couldn't do—that very individual was Dr. Falowski!

It is pretty amazing to look back on your life and see a bigger and better reason why things happen. In retrospect, I see that the path my drunken seventeen-year-old self went down led me to a means of making use of my mistakes. The trauma I went through equipped me with the experience of helping those with no hope. That God would make good come from my foolish mistakes is evident decades later. Even His hand in completing this book is evident as I finally close my writing of it.

A Special Bonus Gift from Dr. Gallagher

Now that you've secured your copy of **Is Your Head on Straight?** you are on your way to learning about a very important yet often overlooked disturbance to your nervous system. Not only will you encounter numerous cases of patients who suffered from neurological insult but you will also discover their miraculous stories of regaining a balanced life.

There are so many drugs to mask the pain of migraines, vertigo, and other ailments, but if the atlas is out of proper alignment, medicine cannot correct the problem. When you finish this book, not only will you know what symptoms are common indicators of this type of injury but you'll also know how to seek the care to correct the problem.

To thank you for your purchase, I have created a special feature with ten tips for a healthier spine. Please visit the following URL and tell us where to send this bonus gift:

http://isyourheadonstraightbook.com/bonus

I am in your corner. Let me know if I can help further.

Here's to getting your or your loved one's head back on straight!

Sincerely yours in the world's greatest health profession,

Patrick Gallagher, DC, BCAO
http://chiropracticfirstnc.com

Appendix A

Chi Stretch

After years of implementing the Chi Running mindset, I became acutely aware of what my body was sensing when I put the method to use and when I did not. Danny Dreyer has given me permission to share what I believe to be a key component of Chi Running, Body Looseners, or what I have coined Chi Stretch. You can find more on this in his book, *Chi Running*.[52] I find that this stretch benefits any activity that requires good, fluid body motion. I do this stretch before golfing, skiing, hiking, and, of course, before every run. Going through the Chi Stretch takes little more than two minutes. The focus is on the ligaments, for the muscles will get their warm up shortly into the run or activity. At marathons, I often see runners sprinting around for their warm up and think, "So this is your first marathon, huh?" When you are going to run for hours and hours, you need to save your fuel. Enough on that, on to the stretch:

Begin with your ankles. In a balanced stance with feet shoulder-width apart, place the toes of one foot on the ground, just behind the other foot. Roll the ankle in circles ten times clockwise and ten times counterclockwise. The ankle should be relaxed, letting the knee do the work. Repeat on the other side.

---

[52] Danny Dreyer and Katherine Dreyer, *Chi Running: A Revolutionary Approach to Effortless, Injury-Free Running* (New York: Fireside, 2009), 98–108. Also see www.chirunning.com.

Focus on knees next. Place your hands on your knees. Now roll your knees in a clockwise motion for ten circles and then counter-clockwise for ten circles.

Loosen the ball and socket of the hips. This is a challenging but important one. Stand up straight with your knees slightly bent. Move both knees together in a clockwise motion and then counterclockwise for ten circles in each direction. Keep your feet on the ground and keep your knees a half-circle out of sync. You can put your palms over the balls of your hip to get a sense of this motion. (Once, within the first tenth of a mile of a half-marathon, I quickly realized that I had failed to do this section of my Chi Stretch. To avoid injuring my hip sockets, I stepped out of the river of runners and did this one part of the stretch while fifty-plus runners passed me by. Still, I did overtake many of them in the ensuing thirteen miles.)

Stretch the ligaments of your pelvic base. Focus on your tailbone, for that is where the ligaments are that you want to stretch. Place your hands on your hips, tilt your pelvis forward, then to the right, backward, and finally to the left. Move through these four directions ten times. Do this both clockwise and counter-clockwise. If you feel like you are belly dancing, that's a good sign.

Stretch the spine. This one I tweaked a little from Dreyer's book. Stand with your feet shoulder-width apart, relax your back, and stretch down toward your feet. Go as far as is comfortable, remain there a second, and come back upright slowly, like going uphill on an old-fashioned rollercoaster, one link at a time. Continue on over the top and extend backward as far as you can comfortably go. Do this three times. From the first to the third time you do this, you should notice an increase in your stretch.

Add a spinal twist. Stand with your feet together, interlock your fingers behind your neck, and rotate your upper body.

When you turn and bend right, look toward your left foot and vice versa on the other side, keeping your elbows out to the sides.

Finally, perform an upper-body shake out. Stand with your feet hip-width apart, step back with one foot, straighten out that knee, and slightly bend the front knee. Focus on your hips while relaxing your upper body. Now twist your pelvis, let your shoulders and arms be like cotton, and just flop side to side in an effortless motion. I like to view this as my core strength showing me what has the power when it comes to full-body motion: it's not my legs nor my arms: it's my core. The stronger my core strength is the greater I can lean forward and let gravity truly push me on my run.

A shout-out to Danny! Although my first three marathons were completed without Dreyer's teaching, thanks to him I have painlessly run twice as many marathons.

Appendix B

Interview with Doctor Roy Sweat

Interviewing Dr. Roy Sweat is like chatting with an old friend. Within minutes of being introduced to him by Patrick by way of a telephone conversation on July 21, 2016, I was laughing and having a wonderful time. As a journalist, I had interviewed thousands of people but had never had such a relaxed, fun time doing so as I did that afternoon.

— Susan Bowmer

By Susan Bowmer and Dr. Patrick Gallagher

At ninety years of age, Dr. Roy Sweat still works six days each week teaching as well as treating patients. Along with his son, Dr. Matthew Sweat, he teaches AO at Life College in Marietta, Georgia, in addition to teaching two weekend courses at the Palmer Institute in Davenport, Iowa. Sherman College of Chiropractic, in Spartanburg, South Carolina, also offers AO courses.

His invention, the Atlas Orthogonal Percussion Instrument, is used by more than 600 chiropractors, 75 percent of which are Board Certified Atlas Orthogonalists, in Spain, Italy, Germany, Japan, England, Dubai, Australia, and the United States.

When asked why patients should seek AO treatment, Sweat said that while studying under B.J. Palmer, he and Dr. John Grostic felt there should be a better way to align patients' heads, necks, and atlases than by hand. "We wanted to create an instrument to do the same thing" because all people are different and the doctors need to be able to give the same care no matter their size or strength. The percussion instrument makes all doctors equal, for the force does not come from the doctor but from the instrument, which is perfectly calibrated to correct the misalignment of the atlas.

The first Atlas Orthogonal Percussion Instrument was built in 1970, and Sweat said, "We have not had a recorded incident of harm" from them. "I don't run down hand adjustments," but with the machine "you can set more minute adjustments and the treatments are constant, not variable as humans are." While B.J. Palmer's method of toggling patients required forty pounds of pressure, by 1947 Sweat and Grostic only needed fifteen. The Atlas Orthogonal Percussion Instrument only uses six pounds of pressure, which Sweat said is "lighter and lighter, making it safer for the patients."

"We take X-rays before and after the procedures to show the difference," he said. "Percussion puts much less force on the patient's atlas. By taking two sets of X-rays, we can show what moved, how much, and which way. AO is the only chiropractic program using percussion."

While adamant about not comparing AO success rates with those of other types of chiropractic care, Sweat said, "In our opinion, it [the percussion instrument] has the ability to accurately and precisely deliver a corrective force to the atlas. There is less physical exertion on the patients and doctors. I'm eighty-nine years old,[53] and with the machine you can't get too tired. The function of the machine is simply pushing a button, not the doctor using his strength. Having the machine makes all doctors equal. You just hit the button and the patients get the

---

[53] Dr. Sweat, currently ninety years old, is still providing atlas orthogonal chiropractic care.

same treatment whether they are in South Carolina, California, Georgia," or anywhere else. Indeed, AO Travel Cards allow patients to "transfer from one state or area to another. They can be adjusted by their new doctor without having to retake the X-rays because all the doctors are using the same instruments," he said. On these cards is the vital information an AO doctor derives from the X-ray to make the precise adjustment. But for a major trauma, like a car accident or fall in which the skull is struck, this information stays the same.

Sweat feels that children should have the same access to AO as adults. "Children are small adults and every bit as important," he said. "Once they have their initial X-rays, those X-rays can be used for the rest of their lives." Shy of an unexpected trauma, this is true. Dr. Gallagher said he learned from Dr. Sweat that once a patient has a major listing of a misalignment, it's always a major—unless a major insult. This means that the way an atlas misaligns is the way it always will, shy of a major trauma.

Sweat calls AO "a conservative program using a scientific approach to chiropractic."

This book would not be complete without giving a shout-out to Dr. Roy Sweat. If it were not for his ability to be such a great teacher, who lives out what he believes, the success stories in which I played a role would not have been possible. As one of my military patients once said, "I think Dr. Sweat is onto something with that atlas work."

Original Text of the Case Study on Baby Liam

Study of Atlas Adjustment and Profound Effect Upon a Baby's Health

Author: Patrick Gallagher, DC, BCAO
Chiropractic First PC
1304 East Ash Street
Goldsboro, North Carolina, 27530
(919) 735-4300

Disclaimers: This is only a single case and I am only stating the clinical findings and outcome of this case. I am not purporting anything beyond that.

Patient's/parental consent to this case study was obtained and is on file.

Key Words: Atlas adjustment, Strep throat, Fever, Otitis media (ear infection), Tracheal constriction.

Introduction

Patient has been brought to the emergency room on a number of occasions with fevers, difficulty in breathing, and ear infections. Treatment consisted of amoxicillin, cortisol, and other medications. They seem to work, yet for only a short time period.

The patient was a twenty-one-month-old male with chief complaints of strep throat, ear infections, a history of fevers, and difficulty in breathing. The patient was presented with a strep throat on his initial visit. By age of twenty-one months, he had had four ear infections and four to five fevers ranging up to 103.8 degrees that lasted up to three days. He also had difficulty in breathing due to his throat being constricted.

History

The child's delivery lasted twenty-four hours, which ended in Caesarian Section. At six months of age, while at a day care center, the baby was dropped off a table onto a concrete floor. He was taken to the emergency room for that injury. It was noted after that injury that the baby would begin to repeatedly hit his head against a wall. The child's pediatrician noted the child was behind in speech development. The child has not slept a solid night through as of March 12, 2014, (about fifteen months) typically wakes up between 1–3:00 a.m.

Examination

A supine leg-length check (face up) showed a difference of a quarter inch with the left side being shorter. Scanning of the upper cervical aspect of the child's neck revealed a tender nodule at C-2 on the left. Leg length became balance with a challenge (stroking the vertebrae in a corrective motion) to the atlas of ASLP (Atlas Superior Left Posterior).

X-rays confirmed the listing.

The patient was diagnosed with cervical subluxation of C-1, ICD 839.01.

Management and Outcome

The first visit on March 12, 2014, the patient had his atlas/C-1 adjusted with a double thumb toggle (thumb over thumb with a little thrust) on a drop head piece (a specially designed cushioned block for the baby that drops a quarter inch with the thrust applied). In the following ten-minute rest period (mandatory for all my atlas patients) the child fell asleep. The child has been seen twice since that first adjustment. The following visit revealed a left ilium/hip subluxation (misalignment) along with C-5 also to the left. His last visit his fourth thoracic and his second lumbar both showed involvement to the left. On both of those visits, his neck scanned clear and his supine leg check showed balanced leg lengths.

Since the first visit, all family members have noticed the child no longer hits his head against the wall. No reports of ear infections or fevers since the first adjustment. He has been consistently sleeping the whole night through, shy one night when he went back to sleep in a few minutes' time. A clinical observation was noted that the child's vocabulary has greatly improved; this too was confirmed by his grandparents.

Discussion

The dramatic changes in the patient tend to be the norm in children that have their atlas/C1 brought back into alignment. It was also noted that the child let out a "coo" the instant his atlas was adjusted. This was noted in another young child adjustment with a similar outcome. If a child has his atlas out of proper alignment, the above symptoms of *otitis media* and fevers are common symptoms of that neurological insult.

Glossary

Acupuncture—A key component of Chinese medicine in which thin needles are inserted into the body, generally for pain relief.

Atlas (C-1)—The smallest bone in the cervical spine, which supports the skull and surrounds and protects the brain stem.

Atlas Neuro Vascular Syndrome (ANVS)—The negative effects on the neurological and vascular systems when the atlas is displaced from a neutral position.

Atlas Orthogonal (AO)—A chiropractic technique specialty focusing on the atlas, which uses a percussion instrument to correct the atlas misalignment.

Atlas Superior Left Posterior (ASLP)— A description of the direction in which an atlas has misaligned.

Audiophobia—Fear of sound.

Axis (C-2)—The largest bone in the cervical spine, the second bone down from the skull.

Board Certified Atlas Orthogonalist (BCAO)—A professional distinction for chiropractors who utilize the atlas orthogonal (AO) technique. Requirements for certification include completing four seminars on basic AO and four seminars on advanced AO, submitting pre- and post-care X-rays to prove that they can perform the technique, and passing a written examination.

Brain Injury Association of North Carolina (BIANC)—An organization in North Carolina with the mission of addressing the needs of the state's brain injury survivors and helping to prevent brain injuries.

Cauterized—Surgically burned.

Cerebral spinal fluid (CSF)—A watery cushion that surrounds and protects the brain, spinal cord, and meninges by absorbing shocks to these areas.

Chiropractic—A healing profession that was founded in 1895; D.D. Palmer coined the term from the Greek *chiro*, meaning "hands," and practic, meaning "practice," or "operation."

Homeostasis—A state of equilibrium necessary for optimal body function.

Innate intelligence—Inborn intelligence that is responsible for the organization, maintenance, and healing of the body. Once interference is removed from the nervous system, innate intelligence can heal the body.

Mastoidectomies—A surgical operation to remove part or all of the mastoid process.

MRI (magnetic resonance imaging)—A medical imaging technique that is used to take internal pictures of the anatomy and the body's physiological processes.

Optic neuritis—Inflammation of the optic nerve, can be caused by multiple sclerosis, which can lead to complete or partial blindness.

Otitis media—An ear infection involving the middle ear.

Photophobia—Fear of light.

Primary sclerosing cholangitis (PSC)—A chronic or long-term disease that slowly damages the bile ducts, which in turn causes the development of cirrhosis or fibrosis of the liver.

Temporomandibular joint (TMJ)—A joint formed by the lower jaw and temporal bone of the skull, inflammation of which can cause mild to severe pain.

Toggling adjustment—Manipulation by hand that is done at a very high speed.

Traumatic brain injury (TBI)—The result of a sudden trauma to the head that causes damage to the brain.

Vertigo—Dizziness or a feeling of motion when standing, sitting, or lying still.

About the Author

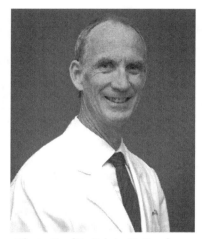

Photo Credit: Calvin N. Sanders,
C&B Photography LLC

Dr. Patrick Gallagher, DC, BCAO, has the inside scoop on traumatic brain injuries. After enduring a horrific motorcycle accident that left him in a coma for eleven days, by God's grace he recovered and discovered from that event his calling to become a chiropractor.

He has a passion for reaching those who are also traumatized in an assortment of ways. Many have been led to believe that conventional medical intervention is the only avenue to well-being, but Dr. Gallagher has learned first-hand the importance of proper head alignment, which allows the body to function the way it was created to be.

Dr. Gallagher is one of about six hundred doctors worldwide who is board certified in atlas orthogonal chiropractic, and he has been applying this special procedure to make miraculous changes in the lives of his patients for the past seventeen years.

Made in the USA
Columbia, SC
24 September 2017